Magic Mushrooms

The Beginner's Guide to Growing Magic Mushrooms

(How to Cultivate and Grow Magic Mushrooms With Psylocibin)

Fernando Quimby

Published By **Andrew Zen**

Fernando Quimby

Magic Mushrooms: The Beginner's Guide to Growing Magic Mushrooms (How to Cultivate and Grow Magic Mushrooms With Psylocibin)

ISBN   978-1-77485-986-5

No part of this guidebook shall be reproduced in any form without permission in writing from the publisher except in the case of brief quotations embodied in critical articles or reviews.

Legal & Disclaimer

The information contained in this ebook is not designed to replace or take the place of any form of medicine or professional medical advice. The information in this ebook has been provided for educational & entertainment purposes only.

The information contained in this book has been compiled from sources deemed reliable, and it is accurate to the best of the Author's knowledge; however, the Author cannot guarantee its accuracy and validity and cannot be held liable for any errors or omissions. Changes are periodically made to this book. You must consult your doctor or get professional medical advice before using any of the suggested remedies, techniques, or information in this book.

Table Of Contents

Chapter 1: Psilocybin Cubensis "Magic Mushrooms _____ 1

Chapter 2: Psilocybin In The Treatment Of Cluster Cerebral Disease _____ 35

Chapter 3: Help For Mushroom Poisoning _____ 62

Chapter 4: Listing Of The Most Commonly Used Types Of Mushrooms _____ 110

Chapter 5: Mycology: Growing Magic Mushroom _____ 153

Chapter 6: Health Mushroom Benefits 159

Chapter 7: Effects Of Magic Mushrooms _____ 167

Chapter 1: Psilocybin Cubensis "Magic Mushrooms

It is well-known to the vast majority of people that magical mushrooms are wild or cultivated , and contain psilocybin in a small portion of its properties as a naturally-occurring psychoactive, hallucinogenic substance. Psilocybin has been consistently considered among the most well-known psychoactive substances, as per The Substance Addiction and Mental Health Service Administration.

What is Psilocybin?

Psilocybin is a specific psychoactive drug.

Psilocybin is a psychoactive substance that acts by activating serotonin receptors. Most often, they are located within the prefrontal cortex. This area of the brain can affect mood, discernment and perception.

Psychoactive drugs affect other areas of the brain that regulate panic and arousal. Psilocybin does not always trigger active auditory or visual hallucinations. In fact, it alters the way those who use tranquilizer see objects and others who are in their state.

The dosage of the medication as well as past experiences and expectations about the way in which the experience will take form can all affect the effects of psilocybin.

Once the gut inhales and consumes psilocybin the body transforms it into the chemical psilocyn. The hallucinogenic effects of psilocybin typically occur within 30 minutes of the time of intake and last for between 4 to 6 hours.

In certain individuals experiencing changes in their sensorimotor recognition and the fundamental patterns of thinking can continue for quite a long duration.

Psilocybin that is found in Mushrooms is typically brown, tan and small. They are commonly regarded by people who live in nature as botch mushrooms that contain Psilocybin, which is a component of many other poisonous mushrooms.

People typically consume psilocybin in the form of an infusion of tea that is fermented, or make it with food to mask its unpleasant taste from the mouth. Dried mushrooms are crushed by manufacturers into powders, and then made into capsules certain people eat these meals with chocolate.

The strength of a mushroom is determined by:

* The species

* The origin

* developing conditions

* harvest period

* whether one takes them dried or fresh

* The amount of active ingredients found in dried mushrooms is 10 times greater than what is of fresh ones.

Psilocybin is classified as to be a Schedule I tranquilize, which means it is highly likely for abuse and is not current therapeutically accepted treatments in United States.

Although some societies have been known to make use of the stimulant properties of certain mushrooms for decades, psilocybin was the first to be isolated in the year the year 1958 by

Professor. Albert Hofmann, who also discovered lysergic-corrosive diethylamide (LSD).

What to know about MAGIC MUSHROOM Use

* Psilocybe cubensis Magic Mushrooms.'

* It's Addiction

* More Addiction

* Medication Use

* Psychedelic drug

* Cocaine

* Heroin

* Pot

* Meth

* Rapture/MDMA

* Opioids

* Prescription Medicines

* Use of alcohol

* Addictions Behaviors

* Nicotine Use

• Coping, Recovery and Resilience

* In this Article

* What do Shrooms do?

Common Side Effects

• Signs of Usage

* The Legends as well as Common Questions

* Addiction and withdrawal

* How to get help

Magic mushrooms are usually dried and then consumed as a part of drinks or food, however certain people consume mushrooms that are freshly harvested.

Shrooms, Freedom tops soft, top gold, philosopher's stones, liberties Amani and agaric are just a few of the names that are known to be associated with magical mushrooms.

Classification of Medication: Psilocybin is characterized and is also known as hallucinogens.

The most common adverse reactions include nausea, yawning, feeling tired, psychosis , hallucinogens. They can cause introspection anxiety, paranoia, and apprehension.

HOW DO I IDENTIFY SHROOMS

Dry mushrooms have a rusty brown color with distinct areas of off-white. Magic mushrooms are consumed mixed with food or fermented as tea to drink. They are also mixed with tobacco or cannabis, and then smoked.

Liquid psilocybin can also be found and is the naturally occurring hallucinogenic medicine that is found inside liberty tops. The liquid is clearer and darker and is contained in a small vial.

What do MAGIC Mushrooms do?

The magic mushrooms can be described as psychedelic substances that can induce you to feel as well as hear and experience sensations that appear real but aren't. Effects of magical mushrooms however, are extremely influenced and are generally accepted as being and in a large way affected by the factors from the environment.

Psilocin is the transformed version of Psilocybin that is found in Mushrooms and the belief that it alters the levels of serotonin in the brain, leading to a change in perception and a lack of. The effects last between 30 and 1 hour to begin and last for up to 6 hours, which is the same length and amount of time to break it into pieces and released as excreters.

There are numerous factors which influence or affect magical mushrooms, such as dosage as well as weight, age as well as the condition of enthusiasm, the history of mental instability. disorders.

What have researchers and experts said?

Magic Mushrooms are typically sought-after for their tranquil and peaceful reasons. Mushroom is known to have been has been proven to trigger anxiety terrifying hallucinations, fear, and confusion for certain people. In reality, the majority of hospitalizations caused by using enchantment mushroom are related to what's commonly referred to as an "awful experience."

Off-Label or Recently Approved Usages

Magic mushrooms are used for a long number of years to provide both deep and restorative purposes for indigenous people in America as well as Europe.

In 2018 research conducted by researchers at John Hopkins University prescribed reclassification of the drug to Schedule I to Schedule IV altogether to allow medical usage. Research suggests that psilocybin could be used to treat cancer-related mental anxiety, depression, distress nicotine addiction, as well as addiction issues related to drugs.

In the year 2019, Denver moved toward becoming the first known and recognized territory that has been approved to curb violent actions towards shrooms. The city is not permitted to "spend resources to impose criminal sanctions" on individuals who own of the drug.

A ESSENTIAL GUIDE TO PSILOCYBIN MUSSHROOMS

(Magic mushrooms, Shrooms, psilocybin)

P

silocybin mushroom has been utilized in therapeutic settings to treat a variety of ailments and problems, such as bunch headaches, supercritical issues and anxiety, sadness and even fixation.

Psilocybin has been legalized within the two North American urban regions (nuances"Authenticity"), they are "Authenticity") However, they're currently illegal and classified as they are a Schedule I controlled substance in the United States. In the last few days however, be whatever it is believed that both the FDA along with the DEA have let a tiny extremely controlled human to think on the possibility of using them in mental and therapeutic settings.

Keen on microdosing psilocybin mushrooms? Participate in our microdosing training course to increase your knowledge

The Manual to Psilocybin Mushrooms

Psilocybin could be an illegal substance, but we do not encourage or advocate any use for this drug particularly in cases where it is unlawful. In any event we recognize that illegal drug use is a reality and believe that providing effective information that reduces the likelihood of hurt is crucial to protect people. Therefore, this guide is intended to safeguard the health of those who decide to make use of the drug.

System

Psilocybin mushrooms (AKA enchantment and mushrooms) is the name that is given to the development that contains Psilocybin, which is a common hallucinogenic substance. There are more than 180 kinds of such mushrooms, which contain psilocybin or its subordinate psilocin. Psilocybin is a psilocybin-related mushroom with a lengthy and storied history of use in Mesoamerica in a variety of otherworldly and strict customs . They currently one of the most widely known recreational hallucinogens within Europe, the United States and Europe.

STATS AND HISTORY

The archeological evidence found in the desert proves that psychedelic mushrooms were utilized by humans for many years. Mushrooms have been mentioned in the art of prehistoric times across many diverse geographical regions. Most of the time, they're considered to be purely symbolic, typically when they are used in ceremonies of right of passage. In the event that our ancestors did indeed use mushrooms, this profound experience could have had an impact on the ancient culture in all aspects, from religion to art to the values of society that guided the daily routine.

Others have gone more. Terence McKenna, for one presented the "Stoned Ape Hypothesis," positing that the earliest humans, or prehuman primates ate mushrooms, resulting in evolutionary benefits, including improvements in intelligence. It is important to note that this theory is viewed with suspicion by the scientific community, as the fact that McKenna's ideas are not supported by evidence to support them.

As far as pre-Columbian times go The most extensive and thorough information was gathered through research conducted by the Aztec as well as Mayan communities of Mesoamerica especially located in Mexico as well as Guatemala. After the conquer of these regions in the 15th and 16th centuries of years The Spanish banned the use of hallucinogenics by indigenous peoples, judging it as barbaric and un-Christian practice. However, indigenous shamans resisted Spanish laws in obscurity for more than 400 years to protect their cultural heritage with these well recognized mushrooms.

The first known and trustworthy stories in the world of intoxication" using enchantment fungi came in 1799, when four kids were fed accidentally Psilocybe semilanceata, which is a type of hallucinogenic fungus.

The famous Swiss scientist Albert Hofmann (who organized LSD) first isolated psilocybin within the lab in the year 1957. Psilocybe Mexicana which is a kind of mushroom that is found within Central America. After a few years it was artificially created simply because. Gordon Wasson, previous unfortunate propensity-driven leader of J. P. Morgan and Company Evidently, he had an interest which morphed into a fascination with psilocybin fungi. In 1955, he took an trip in Oaxaca, Mexico, to meet Maria Sabina, an individual of an indigenous Mazatec Indian clan and a mushroom shaman. She showed Wasson to psilocybin as well as spiritualist shamanism. When he first went on a mushroom excursion the man announced his inclination "as as if his spirit was being sucked from your body."

Wasson was able to kick-start the improvement of hallucinogenic mushrooms in the West when, in the year 1957, Time Magazine appropriated his photo paper entitled "Looking at the Wonder Mushroom," in which Wasson detailed his experiences.

After studying of the experiences of Wasson and following going to Oaxaca to see psilocybin fungi to test for them, Timothy Leary and Richard Alpert who were experts at Harvard University started an experiment called the Harvard Psilocybin Project, which clearly, saw the two men immediately terminated at this point on. The two did what every scholastic who was unemployed could have accomplished in the year 1962 when they started an euphoric development. The psychedelic mushroom was quickly accepted into the counter-culture of the 1960s.

The year 1971 saw the first time that psilocybin became listed in the United Nations' Convention on Psychotropic Substances as a Schedule I sedate in the United States, making it illegal for any reason. In any case, psilocybin is not included in the UN appearance, which, until today, allows nations that have endorsed the event (basically an agreement) to control the mushrooms which normally contain psilocybin, as they think appropriate. Today, psilocybin is prohibited in many nations, however there are some exceptions.

In the past couple of years, administration bodies like FDA and the DEA or FDA have relaxed the rules for using psilocybin for controlled research trials more than any other psychoactive. Energizing new research on psilocybin as both a therapeutic instrument and as a part of individual/otherworldly improvement strategies has been published and continues to be done today.

Current usage

Psilocybin mushrooms are among the most commonly used psychedelics in those aged 34 and under.

A report from the past of 409 college students from the American northeast found that nearly 30% of the students that were interviewed had used psilocybin mushrooms at least three times.

A study conducted by the NSDUH conducted in 2010 shows that, when compared with other substances, psychedelics -- which are in agreement with the NSDUH comprises LSD, PCP, peyote mescaline and psilocybin fungi and MDMA (ecstasy) --were used by approximately 1.2 percent of the population of people aged 12 years old or older in the preceding month. Incredibly, the term "psychotherapeutics" is reported to be frequently used in a manner that is almost three times higher than hallucinogenics.

Surveys conducted in 12 EU regions found that between the ages of 15-24 are using enchantment mushrooms from less than 1% to 8percent.

In the UK nearly 340,000 people between the ages of 16 and 59 consumed enchantment-based mushrooms in the most recent year of 2004/2005. This was just prior to when they were declared unlawful in the UK.

Optimize your microdosing efforts

Are you stressed about having too much to drink measurement, not doing it correctly or losing control of your experiences?

HOW DO I MICRODOSE

PHARMACOLOGY

The main hallucinogenic ingredient found in hallucinogenic mushrooms is called psilocybin. The portion that controls predisposition the effects of dried enchantment mushrooms typically falls within the 0.2-0.5g area, but it differs across clients. A moderate portion of the 1-2.5g area, taken orally, typically results in an excursion lasting between 3 and 6 hours.

Psilocybin is transformed into psilocin. Both of that give the impression of being similar to one another in the way they transmit hallucinogenic effects. Psilocybin is about a hundred times less revolutionary than LSD and is a lot less secure than mescaline.

Psilocybin as well as its derivative, psilocin are primarily associated with serotonin receptors inside the brain. It is particularly arousing attraction to 5-HT (serotonin) subtype 2A of receptors. In rodents psilocybin shows an unreliable connection with receptors located in the focus point area.

What can you expect?

A typical trip with an average portion of the enchantment mushroom (1-2.5g) is characterized by an increased intensity of intense experiences with increased attention to detail, as well as altered psychological functioning in the form of "hypnagogic experiences" that is, a temporary state that combines attentiveness and relaxation. It is typically described as a dreamlike state, and brain studies have shown that a trip to the mushroom can be neurologically similar to dreams.

Perceptual changes, such as dreams and synaesthesia (mixing sensory modalities, e.g. hearing colors, taste sounds) as well as intense changes and a distorted sense of time, are typical of a trip to the mushrooms. The effects are usually observed within 1 - 1.5 hours after ingesting the psilocybin portion of the mushroom.

You'll notice changes in your perception of your surroundings. There could be shifts in your recognition of visuals like the radiances of lights, articles as well as geometric drawings while your eyes are closed.

Your feelings and thoughts may also change. It is normal to experience the feeling of being open to thoughts and emotions that which you, on the whole avoid in your normal daily life. An appreciation and joy with your surroundings, people who surround you as well as your thoughts are not uncommon, as is the feeling of peace and connection with the world.

Feelings of intense intensity are a constant experience both terrible and great. It is recommended that you keep these feelings from way, but instead allow them to follow their own path. A lot of reports that reveal extreme negative feelings also include the feeling of peace and disconnection from them, especially if they tell themselves that emotions will pass quickly.

Physical symptoms vary from person to person and may include changes in the heart rate (up and down) as well as changes in blood mass (up and down) illness, enlarged tendon reflexes, tremors increased pupils and anxiety and problems with growth.

Another study found that psilocybin may cause cerebral discomfort in healthy individuals that may last several days. The subjects did not suffer extreme headaches, regardless and psilocybin can be utilized by some for the treatment of the clinical condition known as chronic cerebral pains (see the practical applications segment).

BAD TRIPS

Anyone who is interested in trying Psilocybin at first is bound to be concerned at some point whether they will experience an "awful experience" with dizzy hallucinations, paranoia that is uncontrollable and reckless behavior are typically among the most frequently-reported concerns. The possibility of having a disastrous experience is real but the risk are minimized by adhering to the six pillars of the hallucinogenic experience. Be prepared and aware of your motives prior to embarking on a psychoactive experience can help you manage the risks.

Dose-based effects.

Note: The effects listed below are not intended to be comprehensive especially at lower portions of levels.

Note: These ranges are only applicable to Psilocybe cubensis, a mushroom. They may apply to other psilocybin-containing species, yet some (for example, P. semilanceata) are more potent than normal.

* Microdose (0.05-0.25 g)

* Improvement in the state of mind

* Reduced stress

* Passionate solidness

* Love, care and peace

• Transparency, self-forgiveness and honesty

* Greater empathy and social ability

* Conversational smoothness

* Relieving chronic conditions like depression, unease and PTSD, ADD/ADHD

* Increased motivation (for instance, to implement positive lifestyle modifications)

* Improved productivity and focus

* Stream states are increased.

* Clearer, more progressively connected thinking

* Increased memory

* Higher faculties

* Enhanced appreciation for work, music and more.

* Increased creativity

* Spontaneity

* Simpler reflection

Increased enjoyment from regular activities and physical activity.

• Unwinding, and increasing awareness of the body

* Increased athletic endurance

* Increased energy in general (without tension or a resulting accident)

* Amplification of the state of mind, either positive or negative

* Slightly effect of sedation

* Hyper states that are conceivably conceivable.

* Possiblely increased neuroticism

* Mini-dose (0.25-0.75 g)

* Mood enhancement, mild emotion or excitement

"Mindfulness," presence and harmony

* Self-forgiveness and acceptance

* Introspective insights

* Reduction in persistent illnesses such as anxiety, despondency as well as PTSD, ADD/ADHD and depression.

* Increased motivation (e.g. to implement positive lifestyle adjustments)

* Flow states that are more pronounced.

* Clearer and more connected thinking

* Better senses

* A greater appreciation of art, music and more.

* Creativity boosted

* Spontaneity

* Easier contemplation

* More enjoyment from regular exercise and daily activities.

Increased awareness of the body

* More energy in waves

" Mild Body High

* Improvement of state of mind, either positive or negative

* A preference for reflection over mixing

* Greater sensitiveness to light

* Very light visuals in the event that there are there is any

* Hyper states that can be imagined.

* Potentially expanded neuroticism

* Tough to center or thought loops

* Some difficulty with task that are subjective

* Anxiety, nervousness or anxiety

* Mingling with distress or difficulty

• Dissatisfaction with dosage (too high for comfort or too low to be "recreational")

* The historical central part (0.5-1.5 g)

* Mind-set enhancement, euphoria or fervor

* Moderate to light visuals (e.g. "breathing" environments)

* Greater compassion

* Conversational ease

* Introspection

* Flow states are increasing.

* New senses

* Improved appreciation of art, music and more.

* Greater creativity

* Spontaneity

* Greater enjoyment from daily activities and physical activity.

* Observing things that are otherwise boring amusing or entertaining

* Increased athletic endurance

Medium body-high

• Clear coming-up and pinnacle and descent

* Exaggeration of mood, either positive or negative

* Modified perception of the sound

* Time contraction or expansion (time moving more slowly or quickly)

* Increased sensitivities to light

* Pupil dilation

* The difficulty of centering or thinking circles or difficult to think about.

* There is a difficulty with certain tasks.

* Inconvenience or difficulty mixing

* Frustration over measurement (at the lower end)

* Moderate portion (2-3.5 g)

* Excited or strong euphoria

* Peaceful feeling

* An experience that is magical and a feeling of wonder

* Life-changing philosophical or inner-reflective ideas

* A broader stream of ideas

* Creativity boosted

* Increased senses

* A greater appreciation for the arts, craftsmanship and so on.

* Finding things that aren't normally interesting or clever

* High body strength

• Clear coming-up and pinnacle and descent

* Exaggeration of emotions regardless of whether they are terrible or great

* Visuals that are open and closed (e.g. patterns and auras)

* Synesthesia

The term "time dilation" or "removal" refers to the process of (time passing more slowly or more quickly)

* Sedation

* Unusual physical sensations

* Sensitivity towards light

* Wide pupil enlargement

* Enthusiastic yawning

* Perplexity

* Disorientation

* Anxiety and fear ("awful" experiences)

* Difficulty in task-related tasks that are subjective

* Unsteadiness

* Nausea

* Mega portion (5+ g)

* A strong euphoria or excitement

* Awe-inspiring experience, awe-inspiring feelings and of wonder

* Life-changing philosophical or contemplative ideas

* Ego death

• Increased flow of ideas

* Greater innovation

* Better senses

* Finding things that are not commonplace amusing or interesting

* Extremely strong body high

* A clear come-up, peak and come-down

* Enhancement of emotions regardless of whether they are good or bad

* Very reliable open- and closed-eye dreams (e.g. Recollections popping up)

* Audio-visual hallucinations involving material

* Synesthesia

* Time becomes useless

* Thought circles

* Sedation

The sensations are unique and physical and altered perception of physical shape

* Sensitivity towards light

* Very large pupil dilation

* Compulsive yawning

* Disarray

* Disorientation

* Motor functions that are impaired (sitter is recommended!)

* A strong dread and unease (extreme "awful excursion" experiences)

Extreme difficulty with cognitive tasks

* Dizziness

* Queasiness

* Headaches and lightheadedness.

Legends/Myths

" Magic Mushrooms can cause bleeding in the brain or stomach bleeding. Kidney Failure"

The term "draining cerebrum" is interpreted as a discharge, stroke or aneurysm. There isn't any evidence of this occurring frequently as a result of eating Psilocybin mushrooms. Nor does there exist any evidence to suggest that the mushrooms can cause stomach bleeding. A study from 1981 found those two prevalent ailments associated with mushrooms included prolonged understudies and overly sensitive reflexes. Other studies on composition have revealed no difficulties with the use of mushrooms in healthy individuals.

Concerning kidney problems it's an issue of distinctive proof from the mushroom. The hallucinogenic species of mushroom Psilocybe semilanceata does not cause kidney problems.

However, the mushrooms belonging to the family of Cortinarius frequently mistakenly identified as P. semilanceata. They are harmful to kidneys.

"Shrooms can cause you to get crazy."

Scientists have drawn parallels between psilocybin-related trips and maniacal-like scenes similar to schizophrenia-related ones but in most cases, it is a short (consequently the term "trip"). Even those that are taken to the emergency rooms after taking the enchantment mushroom return to their normal mental and physical state within the span of a few hours. In actuality, an ongoing vast study by the researchers found less risk of depression and suicidality in the most exemplary hallucinogenic (LSD or enchantment based mushrooms, and others.) consumers.

There is no evidence to suggest that the underlying mental health problems could be worsened by use of hallucinogens. However, this is an opinion held by a variety of researchers. In all likelihood, if you've had a history of dealing with mental disease (particularly schizophrenia) it is advised to stay away from psychedelic drugs.

31

"Shrooms are harmful."

The question of whether this myth can be considered "genuine" and not, it depends upon your definition of "dangerous." If you plan to create a substance that is toxic, causes to a state of intoxication, alters the state of your brain, and causes a change in your body's physiological and, in that case certain, enchantment mushroom can be harmful. If that's the case, then all drugs are dangerous such as tobacco, alcohol and caffeine, and many others. A less defining definition of a substance that is dangerous, in any event, will not have any effect on mushrooms in any way.

It is crucial to distinguish the harm caused by mushrooms from non-hallucinogenic species as well as "inebriation" by hallucinogenic species. Charm mushrooms aren't harmful and do not cause any serious health issues. There are non-hallucinogenic species which could make you physically sick, and they can be harmful enough to cause severe damage or, in extreme circumstances, death. The legitimate proof of differentiation between mushroom species in this way is extremely important.

Improve your microdosing endeavors

Are you stressed about excessively, not estimating precisely, or losing the control over your experiences?

Learning how to microdose

Very helpful USE

Numerous preclinical preliminary studies in between the years 1960 and 1970 indicated the potential of psilocybin and various hallucinogenics for treating diverse disorders, such as headaches caused by bunches as well as state of mind issues and addiction.

When the federal government introduced the psilocybin plant as one of the Schedule I composition during the 1970s, the investigation into its effects on the body has been to all practical purposes ineffective since the time of its renaming. Numerous indirect studies of the effects of psilocybin's regenerative properties have at last caught the attention of experts in medicine and researchers, who have increased funding for the scientific study of hallucinogenic mushrooms as well as research institutes like for example, MAPS, The Beckley Foundation and the Johns Hopkins Center for Psychedelic and Consciousness Research.

Chapter 2: Psilocybin In The Treatment Of

Cluster Cerebral Disease

The luster migraine is often considered to be the most threatening and irritating type of cerebral discomfort to suffer from. They're more intense than headaches that cause cerebral pain however they rarely persist for long. Nighttime ambushes are often more complex and intensive than daytime cerebral pain cluster attacks, but both interfere with the lives of individuals generally.

There are no formal research has been conducted to discuss the potential treatment benefits of psilocybin in treating headaches. However, numerous reports from anecdotes have attracted interest from the therapeutic community. In the early 2000s, medical experts began to pay attention to Psilocybin and LSD as potential treatments for the condition known as cluster cerebral disorder following several of patients reported a decrease in their conditions due to recreational hallucinogenic use (and later self-medication).

One current survey has found that psilocybin may be more effective in the treatment for headaches caused by clusters than the current medications available nearly 50% of sufferers mentioning this drug as an effective treatment in depth.

Psilocybin as a treatment for anxiety and mood disorders.

The evidence from the past has suggested the use of psilocybin (and other hallucinogenics) as a remedy for problems with the mind such as anxiety and wretchedness. Doctor. James Fadiman has been gathering these stories for a long time in the past, and a good portion of them have been positive.

The government has allowed certain small, extremely controlled studies to focus to the effectiveness of psilocybin in dealing with temperament issues. The year 2011 saw a brief trial was conducted to examine the impact of psilocybin in reducing depressive symptoms and tension at the end of life in terminally ill patients. The participants in the study were diagnosed with propelled organ malignancy as well as an underlying diagnosis of anxiety or stress associated with their illness. The researchers observed massive improvements following psilocybin treatment in the levels of anxiety and depressive symptoms for up to one-half year following the initial. This study is now granted the Phase II approval by FDA.

Beginning late, a renowned research team in London is conducting a study that suggests psilocybin might be utilized to treat serious anxiety. 12 patients were treated with two doses from psilocybin (one low, and the other high) along with mental aid. Over the course of a few weeks after the next dose of treatment, the distress scores were down and down in nearly every patient and 8/12 showed no sign of sadness. After a quarter of a year in the future the five patients were depressed, while the remaining seven experienced a decrease in the severity of their depression to "Serious" down to "Mild or moderate."

Treatment with psilocybin has also been observed to reduce the symptoms of obsessive-compulsive Disorder (OCD) through an investigation of a few patients who did not respond to conventional serotonin the reuptake inhibitor (SRI) non-silent treatment. In this investigation the patients all showed decreased OCD reactions ranging from 23 percent and 100 percent.

PSILOCYBIN In The Treatment of ADDICTION

It is believed that "exemplary hallucinogenics" were employed in preclinical research trials to treat addiction during the 1950s and 1960s with promising outcomes. But, since the majority of these psychedelics were banned within the US and the majority of Europe and the world, research into their use in a therapeutic context was largely stopped. Recent research has shown a renewed interest in the use of psilocybin and various hallucinogenics to treat addiction.

Psilocybin as part of a plan to treat addiction has shown promise in the treatment of alcohol abuse through non-clinical tests in ongoing study in 2015.

The substance is also believed to be a possible source to help people quit smoking tobacco. In a study currently in progress two to three treatment sessions using psilocybin as part of a larger cognitive-behavioral treatment program for smoking cessation had an 88% success rate in reducing smoking among the subjects (12 from 15 participants). Contrast this with regular methods for smoking cessation that have high results (e.g., patches, gum cold turkey. have a 35% of success.

Does PSILOCYBIN RE-FIRE THE BRAIN?

Certain researchers are beginning realize that many positive effects of psilocybin's use on mental health issues could result from its capability to reset the control system of the cerebrum. This is known as D Psilocybin in the Treatment of Mood and Anxiety Disorders

The evidence from the past has suggested Psilocybin (and other hallucinogens) as a remedy for mental issues like anxiousness and wretchedness. The Dr. James Fadiman has been collecting these stories for quite some time in the past, and many of these have been positive.

N which is also known as the default Mode Network which has been associated with depression and other disorders of temperament when it is excessively active. Psilocybin has been proven to dramatically lower the activity of DMN that has recently been linked to its antidepressant effects.

In the early stages of studies in which hallucinogenics were administered to healthy adults in strong conditions, several participants discovered long-lasting, profitable changes as aspect of their personality, their behaviour, as well as their traits and behaviors. In lieu of precise evaluations have confirmed these findings since people often report greater enthusiasm for the arts, work and nature, as well as greater resilience to others and a more creative and creativity after taking a trip with mushrooms.

Further studies have also confirmed the early findings. Around 40% of the participants in several research centers' investigations into Psilocybin showed positive, long-term effects on fashion perception and their relationship with the natural world.

A different study in 2011 revealed over a year following an solitary exposure to psilocybin , transparency character percentages were not lowered for the study subjects. The experts believe that the remarkable experience is a constant awards.

Legality

Psilocybin is illegal in a number of countries, but their legal status is a possibility in some locations. In the Netherlands due to an escape clause that is legal that allows for the purchase of "charm truffles" with psilocybin in them and not violate the laws. Psilocybin is legal to be found in certain structures in Brazil as well as Jamaica, the British Virgin Islands, Jamaica and the Netherlands.

The United States, while it's illegal at the federal level, psilocybin mushroom were thought to be as legal to cultivate and were in use (so so far) not been dry) been in New Mexico in 2005. In 1978 the Florida exclusive court ruled that the purchase of wild psilocybin mushrooms was legally valid until the state's administration declares something different. There are no Florida law has been passed since then to regulate the collection of wild-picked psilocybin-containing mushrooms.

On May 7, 2019, residents in Denver, CO, cast an election to legalize the psilocybin mushroom. It's now not an offence for people over 21 to possess them for personal use. This doesn't mean they're authentic however. If you're found selling or for the major part, distributing psilocybin mushroom and in all likelihood making the mushrooms, you may currently face criminal charges. In addition, the law is unchanged throughout Colorado, at all times until the next time.

In June of that year, Oakland, CA, adopted their own amendment. Board members threw out a vote form that was able to remove the criminalization of not only psilocybin but also the entire range of "entheogenic plants" with indoleamines and tryptamines and Phenethylamines. In Denver this is only applicable to those aged 21 and over. In addition, it does not apply to substances that are derived from parasites or plants such as, LSD. Be that as it may, not at all like in Denver, it also decriminalizes (or rather deprioritizes for law execution) the improvement and circulation of the predefined hallucinogenics--which include psilocybin mushrooms.

Outside of three states the spores of psilocybin mushroom are legally permitted to be used throughout the United States as the spores aren't containing psilocin or Psilocin synthesized substances that are specifically controlled by law enforcement agencies. However although the spores have legality and produce mushrooms from seeds is still considered an illegal development.

A few important things you need to think about when you are thinking about Magic Mushrooms. Psilocybin is found in many types of mushrooms like Psilocybe mexicana. Psilocybe Mexicana is the mushroom that psilocybin's first isolated.

Psilocybe Mexicana, also known as a magical mushroom.

At first glance, Psilocybe cubensis doesn't look particularly mystical. In reality, the name that is logically associated with this tiny, dark-colored, white mushroom is "bare head" fitting with the species' relatively unassuming appearance. In any case, those who have taken a bite from P. cubensis claim that it alters the reality of the person.

The mushroom is among more than 100 species of plants that contain mixtures that are known as psilocin and Psilocybin that are psychoactive substances and can cause dreams, happiness, and other trippy experiences. They "magic mushroom" have for a long time, been utilized throughout Central America under strict administrations and are now in the shadow market in pharmaceuticals within the United States and different nations that view them as controlled substances.

Self-improvement

What is it that makes a small, unassuming mushroom alter the brain so completely? Find out the bizarre details of the'shroom.

THE MUSHROOM AND ITS LINKAGE TO THE BRAIN

MUSSHROOMS HYPERCONNECT THE BRAIN

The psilocybin-based blends can give users the "mind-dissolving" sensation, however it's exactly the opposite. psilocybin improves the cerebrum's networks according to a Oct. 2014 research. Researchers from King's College London examined 15 individuals to gain an understanding on their mental sifting experience using a functional magnetic resonance imaging (fMRI) device. They conducted the test once following the ingestion of the magic mushrooms, and again following the administration of an untrue treatment. The mind accessibility maps that were emerging showed that, being influenced by the medication, the cerebrum regulates the movement of different regions that aren't normally connected. This change in reality could be the reason for the awe-inspiring expression that people who use the mushroom experience in the aftermath of taking the sedate the researchers said. They may slow the movement of the cerebrum.

"Shrooms" behave in different ways to affect the mind. Psilocybin is a drug that regulates the neuronal connection called serotonin. In spite of the fact that it's unclear exactly what the effect of this connector is on the cerebrum, scientists have found that the drug is associated with other mind correspondence effects, but it also has a greater the synchronicity.

In one study brain imaging in subjects who took psilocybin demonstrated reduced activity in the areas of data transfer such as the thalamus. It is a brain structure that is located in the middle of the brain. It is believed that a decrease in the activity in regions, like the thalamus could allow information to move more easily throughout the cerebrum because that region is a protective area that normally blocks associations, as per the scientists who came from Imperial College London.

Focal Americans used psilocybin fungi prior to the time that Europeans came to the shores of the New World; the fanciful creatures flourish in subtropical and tropical environments. But, how long did individuals stumble across magical mushrooms?

It's not an easy task to respond however a paper from 1992 in the journal of a shorter length, "Joining: Journal of Mind-Moving Plants and Culture," asserted that stonework in the Sahara that has been in use for 9,000 years shows revitalizing mushrooms. The work in question depicts the masked figure holding a variety of objects that resemble mushrooms. Others depict mushrooms that are positioned behind human figures, possibly as a reference to the fact that they grow as fertilizers. (The mushroom images are also decoded as arrows, blooms or other plant material, but it's unanswered whether people who lived in the early Sahara were using'shrooms.)

Magic mushrooms make Santa's possible Poisonous Mushroom. Two red Amanita Muscaria On Green Moss in the Autumn Forest. The beautiful autumn with Amanita muscaria.

Concerning the subject of fantasies, get ready for a somewhat stale tale of Christmas joy. According to Sierra College anthropologist John Rush Charm mushrooms explain the reasons why children believe that a famous flying person will present them with presents on Dec. 25.

Flood stated that Siberian Shamans would carry the blessings of animated mushrooms to nuclear families every winter. Reindeer were considered to be the "soul beings" from these ancient shamans and the consumption of mushrooms might be able to convince a family with a fantasy that these animals are able to fly. Additionally, Santa's white and red suit is reminiscent of the tones of the species of mushroom Amanita Muscaria, which grows -- wait for it -- evergreen trees. But, despite the fact that it looks like a mushroom it is toxic to humans.

You're thinking that you've had a disastrous outing? Do not be stressed. Many anthropologists aren't attracted by the Christmas-related stimulant relationship. However, they are also equally convinced, as Carl Ruck, a classicist at Boston University, revealed to Live Science in 2012: "from the beginning one is convinced that it's absurd however it's certainly not."

'Shrooms may change individuals unexpectedly

A happy lady out in the sun.

The analysts say that a couple of things could alter someone's personality in adulthood, but magic mushrooms may be one of them in some way.

A study from the past found that following a single dose of psilocybin users were moved towards becoming more open to encounters with new people at any time from up to 14 years. This is an incredible change that is steady. People who have open-minded characters are more creative and engaged in their work. They also they value curiosity and feelings.

The reason for this change creates the impression that it is the effects of psilocybin on emotions. The reasons for the shift appears, from all indications to be the impact of psilocybin on the way people feel. People describe mushroom trips as awe-inspiring experiences and express feelings of satisfaction and a sense of connection to others as well as their environment. The extraordinary experiences seem to be a bit distant. (In those tests experts went to great efforts to make sure that the participants didn't experience "awful excursions," as certain individuals react to psilocybin and experience a high vomiting, nausea, and a rash of vomiting. Participants were kept in a space with no music and a calm environment.)

Mushrooms kill fear

A man skims off a slope wearing the help of a harness.

Another peculiar symptom associated with magic mushrooms is that they take out fears. A study that is ongoing of mice revealed that when psilocybin was injected and psilocybin, they were more likely to stop their activities when they heard a roar. they could figure out how to join an electric daze that was not working. Mice who were not treated with the drug were continuously free of the disturbance and, in any case, it took a bit longer.

The mice were fed an insignificant amount of psilocybin. experts said they believe this study will yield forward with more information on the way that mushrooms can be utilized to treat mental wellbeing issues among people. For instance, tiny amounts of psilocybin might be investigated as a method to treat post-traumatic stress disorder, experts suggested.

They create their own wind

Close-up of a magical mushroom.

Mushrooms aren't just there to help people get high. They have their individual lives. Additionally, a part of their lives is multiplication. Similar to other parasites, mushrooms reproduce using methods of spores. They move through the air in search of an additional location to make.

In any event, the mushrooms generally reside in protected locations in forested floors, in areas where there isn't a breeze. To help illuminate the issue in spreading their spores certain'shrooms' (tallying their animating Amanita Muscaria) are able to make their case wind. In order to do this, parasites accelerate the rate at which water evaporates off their surfaces, making water vapor in a visible way all around them. The water vapor, in conjunction with the cool air created through evaporation, is attempting to lift the spores. Together both forces can lift the spores as high as 4-inches (10 centimeters) over the mushroom according to an article in the 2013 meeting at the American Physical Society's Division of Fluid Dynamics.

There are a variety of mushroom species

The gathering of mushroom.

In any case the 144 varieties of mushrooms have the psychoactive fixing Psilocybin as stated in an overview of 2005 published in The International Journal of Medicinal Mushrooms. Latin America and the Caribbean contain more than 50 species as well as Mexico alone is home to 53. There are 22 kinds of enchantment mushroom species in North America, 16 in Europe 19, in Australia in the Pacific island region, 15 in Asia and a minuscule four species in Africa.

Experts are testing different ideas with "shrooms"

Recently, scientists have been exploring a variety of things using the use of psilocybin to treat for nervousness, dejection, and other mental problems. The study that was halted for a long amount of time and is but a challenge to follow due to the fact that psilocybin is a Schedule I substance. It is given from the Drug Enforcement Administration (DEA) for its lack of medical use, and has a high possibility of abuse.

In the past however, psilocybin as well as other stimulants were the heart of an energizing educational program. In the 1960s such as Harvard clinical psychologist Timothy Leary and his colleagues conducted various studies with magical mushrooms known as"the Harvard Psilocybin Project. The most famous of these were The Marsh Chapel Experiment, in which participants were treated with either Psilocybin or fake treatment prior to an assembly at the Church. People who received psilocybin would surely report an extraordinary experience. An analysis of the 25 years since 1991 showed that people who received the psilocybin experience felt considerably more peace and joy than they had reported feeling the previous year, a quarter of a year later. Many described this experience as life altering.

"It provided me with the undisputed assurance that there exists a dimension larger than what I am aware of." someone told experts in 1991. "I am aware of the meaning of that. In the end, it was an idea to an actual one. ... It's funny how it has made my experience atypical in that I have realized there is something going on."

Terence McKenna made 'shrooms standard

Leary's hallucinogenic experiments are an element of the legends about flower children, but the person who did the most to introduce magic mushrooms into normal U.S. steady culture was an ethnobotanist, author and author Terence McKenna. He was exploring various ways to experience hallucinogenics from his teenage years, but, in all likelihood it wasn't until a trip in the Amazon in 1971 that he came across Psilocybin mushrooms- the fields they were, outlined by a 2000 article in Wired magazine.

The year was 1976. McKenna as well as his siblings published "Psilocybin: The Magic Mushroom Grower's Guide" an instruction manual to grow Psilocybin mushrooms in your home. "What is described is significantly more confusing than making jam and making jam" McKenna wrote in the introduction to the book.

Animals feel the impact

Psilocybin "shrooms" grow within the natural environment, therefore it is possible that animals other than humans have examined these trippy species. In 2010, British sensationalist media were abuzz about reports that three young goats living in an asylum run in the 1960s. TV in-screen character Alexandra Bastedo had gotten into natural charms mushrooms. The animals purportedly behaved sluggishly as they ate, sat down, and walked around for two days, and took two days to fully recover.

Siberian reindeer also prefer mushrooms that enchant, as revealed in an article from 2009 BBC nature documentary. It's not known if reindeer experience the effects, but Siberian mystics were known to drink the urine of deer that had consumed mushrooms to make an animated background in order to follow strict traditions.

The Common Side Effects

Each psychedelic substance has the risk of triggering emotional and mental issues, and causing catastrophes, while reducing. For young people the charm mushrooms are often as they can be taken in mixture with liquor and other drugs, increasing the physical and mental risks.

The quantity of psilocybin and Psilocin found in any random enchantment mushrooms is dark. Furthermore, mushrooms vary significantly in amounts of psychoactive substance. It is therefore extremely difficult to determine the duration, strength and the type of "trip" one might take part in.

Consuming a shroom can lead to an enjoyable experience that makes the user feel relaxed or sleepy , with a stunning background. This is which is followed by mind-flights or daydreams and a state of euphoria. In the most sceptical of situations Enchantment mushrooms have been observed to trigger spasms.

The symptoms of charm mushrooms may include mental as well as physical effects.

Impacts: psilocybin impacts

Psilocybin can alter the reality of things and create a sense of passionate prosperity.

The effects of psilocybin are typically similar to those of LSD.

This includes altered alteration of time and space as well as extreme changes in the mood and state of mind.

Possible effects of PSILOCYBIN include:

* Euphoria

* peacefulness

* spiritual arousing

* rapid change in emotions

* derealization, also known as the sensation that the world around you isn't real

* Depersonalization, or a dream-like feeling of being detached from the world around you

* thinking that is distorted

* distortion and visual adjustment like coronas of light, and distinct shades

* Large pupils

* dizziness

*languor

* impaired concentration

* weakness in the muscles

Lack of coordination

* body sensations that are unusual

* nausea

* neurosis

* Perplexity

* frightening hallucinations

* vomiting

* yawning

Effects of Psilocybin vary among people, due to variations in the mental state and personality of the user as well as the immediate state of the user.

If the user of recreational drugs has problems with their mental health or has anxiety about using the hallucinogen, they are at the risk of having negative experiences.

The anxiety of mental health is a worrying event that occurs frequently following the use of recreational psilocybin. The symptoms of this anxiety can be as intense tension or a brief psychosis.

Psilocybin as treatment for depression

There is a debate about whether mental health professionals could make use of psilocybin or similar stimulants to treat depression.

Two ongoing studies have examined the use of psilocybin to treat. One investigation looked at the capability of psilocybin for reducing depressive symptoms without reducing the intensity of emotions. The other examined the relationship between positive positive effects and the possibility of psilocybin-inducing fantasies.

Some researchers are studying various therapeutic applications of psilocybinbut they, currently, view the use of psilocybin as illegal and risky.

Physical effects:

* Nausea

* Yawning

* Increased Heart rate, blood weight and temperature

* Shortcoming in Muscle

* Languor

* Inadequate coordination

* Students who are larger

* Headaches

Mental effects:

* Happiness

* Engaging in contemplative (spiritual) encounters

* hallucinations (visual or audio-related)

* Nervousness

* Neurosis

* Frenzy responses

* Unified perception of place, time and the real

* Psychosis.

Further research is required to determine the long-term and lasting negative effect of the magic mushroom however, it has been discovered that people can experience long-lasting changes in their personality, and flashbacks for a while after they have taken mushrooms.

Because charm mushrooms appear to be poisonous Poisoning is another possible risk associated with consuming the drugs. In the case of poisoning, it can lead to extreme illness or organ damage, and even death.

It's also a common occurrence for enchantment mushroom to be polluted. A study of 886 samples that were deemed to be psilocybin fungi that were broken in with the help of Pharm Chem Street Drug Laboratory found that the lone 252 (28 percent) were extremely psychedelic and 275 (31 percent) were typical privately-sourced mushrooms that were bound to LSD or Phencyclidine (PCP) and 328 (37 percent) did not contain any medicine in any way.

Chapter 3: Help For Mushroom Poisoning

If you believe that you or someone you know has eaten a poisonous mushroom, contact poison control at 800-222-122. Take whatever steps you can to avoid having to wait for signs to prove. They are on hand all day long 7 days a week, all year.

The Signs of Utilization

If you know someone who is taking shrooms, they could be agitated or seem nervous or even suspicious. Because of the use of drugs and the effects of it, it's essential to pay attention to any changes in the way they eat and sleep and changes in mindset and personality and social behavior.

STEPS to GROW MAGIC MUSHROOMS

Step 1. Equipment for Magic Mushroom Culture

Stage 2. Preparing the Spore Jars Syringes

Step 3. Mixing Magic Mushroom Substrate

Stage 4. The Filling of Jars with Substrate. Jars with Substrate

Step 5. Getting ready Substrate Jars for Sterilization

Step 6. Sterilizing Magic Mushroom Substrate

Have you ever wanted to create your own enchantment mushrooms , however you're not scared by the complex steps required to create magical mushrooms. This technique is called PF Tek which is one of the simplest methods of cultivation that is able to cultivate a broad range of enchantment mushroom species, especially those belonging to the Psilocybe class.

Make sure you have the following materials available before you begin developing Enchantment mushrooms:

Stage 1

Pressure cooker.

If you don't own one, look at your local thrift shop to find a basic pressure cooker. It is the most important device for making shrooms. If you don't have it, then don't have the ability to clean the substrate and your shroom will not be as efficient as you'd like.

Vermiculite. It is a material that allows the substrate to retain moisture. It is available in small nurseries as well as big home development stores.

Perlite. It can be purchased in the market for plants in addition. These tiny, white particles help to maintain the quality of air and help improve the breath of plants.

Canning containers. 1/2-1/2-quart containers are fine so long as they're wide-mouthed and have an even spread. They are available at any retailer.

Spore Syringe. Spore syringes can be found on the internet or in nearby stores. Find the spore syringe that has the strain you would like to cultivate.

Aquarium or massive Tupperware. It will serve as your humidification chamber. It is possible to purchase an aquarium for just 10 dollars in a used shop.

Nail and mallet. If you don't of yet have this within your home garage buy one today.

Aluminum foil. It is a must to have it in your kitchen cabinet or on your counter. Visit your local market for a few if you don't see any.

Liquor light. This is essential in the cleaning of needles and various substances. Be sure that the alcohol light you use is effective and secure.

The dark-colored flour is a good choice. This can be used as your substrate. This is which the mycelium will build off. Select the highest high-quality open.

Stage 2.

Making Jars for Spore Syringes

Spore syringes provide the most simple and safest method to begin your enchantment mushroom growth. Based on information available online from a variety of sources. Make sure that you purchase from a reputable supplier to guarantee pleasant, undesirable collections.

However, before you are able to use the spore syringe you must set up your holders with an sledge and nail. Take off the top of the holder and set it on the table. Make use of a nail to make four equally spaced gaps around the edges of the cover.

Stage 3.

Mixing Magic Mushroom Substrate

The substrate is what the organism uses as a source of food. Many substances can be utilized as substrate (for instance, sawdust ground coffee, waste) however, psilocybin mushroom grow very well in dark-colored rice.

Blend the following ingredients in the 8-ounce container:

Darker rice flour, 3 cups

Vermiculite 9 cups

3 cups of water,

Some people even include worm castings in the substrate. Worm castings are believed to increase the number of mushroom blooms. It's not a bad idea to give it a try.

Stage 4.

Pouring into with Substrate. Jars with Substrate

After mixing the damp substrate, pour them into containers that hold substrate. Remove any dampness inside and outside of the compartments. Do not pack them tightly. It is important to leave enough space around the containers. You should leave a significant portion of one inch between the surface and the top within the container.

The remainder of the area with vermiculite that is dry to create an blockage between organisms in the air along with the substratum.

Stage 5.

Preparing Substrate Jars for Sterilization

It is now moment to eliminate all pollutants in the storage containers. Imagine this as cleaning the home to allow mycelia to flourish with no difficulty.

Set a square of foil on top, covering the holes in order to protect the container to prevent contamination from the environment. It is best to press it down to form an edging around the top of the container.

Set 3 water crawls in the pressure cooker, and then place them in the same number of containers you can. You can stack them in case you are running out of space, but be aware that some containers might break.

Stage 6.

Sterilizing Magic Mushroom Substrate

Close the cooker, then begin to run it. Continue to hold it until the pressure control or the pressure gauge on top of the cooker begin to shake. This is usually a sign that the container is currently under eleven to 115 PSI based on the brand of manufacture.

Give the compartments time to be sterilized for 60 minutes.

It's best to carry out this process at night to give the containers the chance to cool down over the night. In the morning, you're prepared for the next step.

Stage 7.

The vaccination of your Magic Mushroom Substrate

The term "vaccine" sounds confusing, but it's not. It's the fundamental method of adding spores to sterilized substrates that allow mycelium hooks and grow.

This is the moment that your substrates are invulnerable to pollution, so take care.

Remove the foil and insert the needle from the syringe for spores into the hole you punched prior to.

Use the plunger to introduce typically one mL of the arrangement onto the substrate.

Repeat this process using different openings in the containers until this point, you can replace the foil.

Repeat the process with other containers.

Important step has been completed!

Stage 8.

Let the Substrates inoculated come forth.

Let the mycelium assume control over the substrate through placing them in warm , dull state. The ideal place to put them is the coordinator on top of your refrigerator, or in a box made of cardboard near the perimeter the room. Ideal temperature is 80-86 degrees F. If it isn't possible to keep your temperature within that zone, it may take a bit longer for mycelium to grow.

At this point mycelium is able to absorb an plenty of nutrients and water off the substratum. The primary hairs of mycelium after 3-4 days. Once you've accomplished everything right, the development will fully populate the substrate in three to five weeks.

Stage 9.

Set Up a Fruiting Chamber for Shrooms

There is no need to worry about numerous exhibitions to make an efficient fruiting chamber. The purpose of this chamber is to create an environment that is high in clamminess for mycelium to release fruiting bodies, also known as Enchantment mushrooms! You only need an aquarium that is old or an enormous Tupperware box.

Make the chamber more humid by filling it up with perlite, which was then soaked in an ice-cold bowl for 5-10 minutes. The base of the container, you fill it with wet perlite. This setup allows water to slowly disappear and create a stickiness in the chamber for fruiting.

Place aluminum foil on the area you'll place the cakes on your substrate.

Make sure to cover the chamber completely. It is possible to drill some holes to let air flow. Enchantment mushrooms require a tiny amount of oxygen in order to live.

Step 10.

Cakes for Birth

The next step is to make the cakes pop or to birth them.

It's not as confusing like human births. Cake birthing is a simple procedure that requires taking off the foil and top, then turning it and then giving the container some smacks to release it.

Following the birth take the cake and suck it up in cold water for a full day. This will shock the

71

parasite into releasing the natural product more quickly. Remember that mushrooms contain about 80-90 percent water.

Stage 11.

Waiting to wait for the Flush

Based on the enchantment type you're using it could take between 2 and 3 months for your first flower to be fully creating. The cakes can continue to bloom for 3-4 blooms. In this case, you can submerge them over 24 hours into water in order to rehydrate them and then reactivate the growing mycelium.

Stage 12.

Gathering Shrooms

When you are picking the shrooms, grasp them from the base and press them down. You may also remove them by removing them from their base.

If you are unable to find these 12 stages with precision and you're still fighting to carry magical mushrooms around the globe Don't be a burden. It's not all lost. You can buy packages for developing truffles with enchantment online. These designs are guaranteed to give hallucinogenic truffles within the shortest amount of time possible and with minimal effort.

If you're making mushrooms using PF Tek or creating a unit, be sure to be conscious of your setting. Enjoy your time!

ANOTHER DETAILED STEPS ON HOW TO GROW MUSHROOMS

A small forest comprised of Amazonica mushrooms

Cultivating fresh Magical Mushrooms

The process of creating your own mushrooms similar to the famous Psilocybe Cubensis Panamericana, also known as the legendary Golden Teacher, or the incredible Psicolybe Mckennaii is now at hand and, as you'll discover in the following, the vast majority could have been easier thanks to this useful guide! This guide will provide an easy-to-follow guide to develop magic mushrooms successfully. The mushroom development kits include everything you'll need to reap excellent results in just a few months with no entanglements or risk and also with mushrooms that are packed with the psilocybin. This is something we should all do!

Stage 1:

Unlock the crate and remove the contents: the mushroom making container, the plastic bag as well as the clip. Take off the cover of the plastic compartment. rinse it well using clean water, and then put it away in a suitable place, you'll need it again (you can keep it in the perfect plastic bag with a zip-close like a).

Stage 2:

Put the plastic holder that contains the material (without any cover) into the additional plastic bag. Slide the opening of the pack under the compartment, keeping the gaps in the scale that are scaled down of the plastic sack moving upwards. This ensures that the bag has sufficient air distribution (the open-air compartment is in all likelihood closed, leaving the compartment "wrapped" inside the breathable bag).

The plastic compartment should be placed inside the pack

Stage 3:

When you notice signs that the main mushrooms will appear on the substrate. You can then reposition the sack vertically and upstanding and allowing the sack enough room for the mushrooms to grow. It is important to note that, despite all that we've not used any of them thus yet! If everything is working the main mushroom should to be visible within seven days.

Stage 4:

Place the bag and holder in an area that has sufficient sunshine (not in direct sunlight anyway!) and at a temperature between 18 to 23oC. They grow at temperatures that are higher than 15oC and above 15oC, however 23oC is ideal for bigger harvests. If it is necessary, you can decorate like with a Root with warming mat is great to ensure a constant temperature for the mushrooms, and it's not essential to warm the entire room in which they're being developed. Some people grow their mushrooms in close proximity to a window during summer and place them inside the nursery to be warmed up during the winter months using some 24W T5 fluorescent cylinders. If you want to protect your belongings place everything in an encapsulated tent to protect replicas.

Place the bag in a well-lit location

You could also make use of an incredibly small grow tent

Stage 5:

If you are able to see the fully mature mushrooms, you are able to remove the bag just enough so that you don't create buildups. In the meantime, excessive moisture could influence the growth of the mushrooms. The principal mushrooms must be harvested within seven days of seeing heads that "grows" within the substratum (organize 3.). Make sure you check the dampness and temperature regularly using an accurate thermo-hygrometer.

After just a couple of days we can begin to see the major mushroom species.

Stage 6:

The moment to pick the mushrooms is vital. Take a glance at the top of the fungus and if it's well swollen but the bottom hasn't yet opened enough to let you observe the gills that hold the spores. By then, you've got the best time to collect them. It's essential to take the spores before they open. This leaves the gills unattended and releasing the spores.

Stage 7:

And, here's some good news that you should know... there is a way to reuse the pack of mushrooms without assuming that you will be immunized with fresh spores! It's as simple as that! Simply, you need to harvest each of the mushrooms, then fill the chamber with clean water. This is a system called a virus stun, which encourages the growth of new life within mycelium. This ensures that the substrate is flooded with enough water to produce another crop of mushrooms.

We'll be taking the main shroom down in the near future.

Stage 8:

The holder should be covered with the top that you placed aside in stage 1. Let it sit until 12 hours. After this time is up you can open the other portion of the top to pour out any excess water that is not being absorbed from the surface. Then, once further, but you have to adhere to the directions at the beginning of stage 1. The unit can be reused several times insofar as you're careful and attentive at every step.

Strategies for growing mushrooms

* Always wear fresh gloves that are clean and fresh, or similar

* Make sure to employ reverse absorption, or refine/filtered water.

*Group of Colombian Psilocybes

The sudden changes in humidity or temperature could slow the process of developing mushrooms along with not-ideal value.

If you are using a heating mat, place the bag that contains the unit on top of the cover, and turn the unit on for the initial two days. Within two or three days switch down the heat until you begin to notice those first "buttons" (about the time of seven days) At that point, you are able to turn it back on by opening the bag a bit to avoid a build-up.

As long as you can dry them the effects of the mushroom will decrease as time passes.

Heat degrades psilocybin rapidly. If you want to store the mushrooms dry them, then put their vacuum-packed jars within an air-tight refrigerator.

Mushrooms were not collected until too late

Mushrooms harvested at optimal minute

In the ideal scenario, we've demonstrated clearly how to cultivate these mushrooms. As you can see, it's extremely simple and you can use the kit several times, resulting in multiple harvests out of every kit. Drop us your comments or questions in the comments section below. We'll be happy to answer.

Happy growing and reaping!

Develop these Mushrooms at home The pros and cons.

Magic mushroom consumers have a variety of choices for techniques for development. Easy and quick? Have an MycoMate The Golden Teacher! Are you interested in starting with scratch?

The Mycelium Grow Units

* Growing magical mushrooms right from scratch

* Grow units that do not contain mycelium

To make it an easy-to-read to you, let us walk through a pros and cons checklist!

Mycelium Grow Kits

Magic Mushroom grow kit. Mycelium Magic Mushrooms Grow Kits are designed specifically to make it accessible and enjoyable for everyone.

With a ready-to-use substrate that is infused with magic mushroom and spores, these packs are "prepared to create."

There is no immunization, or hatching!

Spores are just beginning to develop into mycelium and have colonized the structure of the development unit.

The grow units are nothing less than difficult to operate they provide precise results and provide clear directions.

MycoMate or Freshroom

MycoMate Excellent and reliable It requires more effort and focus on developing, and seems to last for the longest time.

FreshMushroom XP: The new prominent grow pack, the least demanding of guidelines that are perfect for busy individuals, features an incredibly white coating around the base.

Strains

Mycelium grows kit. Each brand comes with its own collection of psilocybe cubenis cultivars. Simple and flexible? And shocking? Fantastic teacher, Mazatapec, or Pes Amazon! Incredible stimulating background? Mexican and McKennaii!

Each strain is unique in their own unique way and require a certain amount of expertise.

Pro's

Delicate and clean

Simple and ideal for newbies

The easiest method to grow magical mushrooms at home is to grow them yourself.

Con's

Limited to one type of cultivation.

Experienced cultivators will require more options to modify cultivating methods.

In addition, the same is applicable to alternative cultivation conditions.

Cons

There's a learning curve. It takes some time and time to master how to make claims cakes.

* These need to be developed from scratchand takes longer than myecelium for it to develop

The working environment should be completely sterile and any contamination can sabotage the entire procedure.

* Brilliant Student spore Syringe 20ml

* Photograph Golden Teacher spore syringe 20ml. Golden Teacher may be referred to by its name,

due to the darker color and gold that the caps. It is the Golden Teacher...

* McKennaii spore vial

Photograph McKennaii spore vessel. It is the Mckennaii Cubensis spores were named for the famous psychonaut and expert Terrence Mc...

Are you curious to learn more about the next stage of cultivation? Take a look at the grow kits with no mycelium!

Alongside magical mushrooms, you can cultivate medicinal and edible mushrooms by using the Kilo Kit as well as an Fast Fungi. Equally exciting is making your own truffles at home using The Underground Kit.

Growth Kit with Mycelium Not Included

Pro's

* In the end, it's cheaper that Mycelium Grow Kits. Kilo Kits Kilo Kit may cost more but it will also produce more.

* The shelf lives of grow kits that do not contain mycelium is more than Mycelium Grow Kits.

It's easier than beginning from scratch. Also, faster and cleaner.

Spores can be legally obtained in numerous countries, for research purposes. In addition, the same is applicable to various types of substrates.

Con's

* There's a small learning curve. It takes some time and time to get familiar with the process of brooding and immunization.

* There is no power over the components that make up the substrate.

* The work environment must be completely clean Any contamination could impact the entire process.

What's your inclination?

If you're new to gardening and would prefer not to spend time on complicated arrangements, you can use the Mycelium Grow Kits.

If you want to be the chef's king as the most sought-after gourmet expert managing every fixing in the recipe starting with no preparation is the most effective strategy.

In addition, if you require something that is in between or you want to move up to a higher level Mycelium Grow Kits the Grow Kits that do not contain Mycelium are the perfect choice for you.

Different types of mushrooms

What are the most popular Sorts Of Magic Mushrooms?

* Psilocybe mushrooms

* Conocybe mushrooms

Copelandia/Panaeolus mushrooms

* Galerina mushrooms

* Inocybe mushrooms

* Mycena mushrooms

There is a wide variety of mushroom species in the air. For instance, the Psilocybin mushrooms have gained the most attention for their psychedelic effects. Do you know there are a variety of kinds of magic mushrooms that produce hallucinogenic effects?

This book outlines the different kinds of stimulant mushrooms, their areas of distribution effect, as well as the distinct features. This book should give you the necessary information to know before you embark on a quest for the magic mushrooms.

Psilocybe mushrooms

Psilocybe is a kind of mushroom that is most well-known for their psychoactive blends including psilocin, psilocin and baeocystin.

The most common types of mushrooms that take spot in this category typically tiny, followed by their small-to-medium tops, a darker or yellow color, and a spore print which ranges from dark-colored lilac up to light-purple. Magic mushrooms are also known to cause be harmful when employed.

20 hours after taking Psilocybe cubensis for 20 hours, one could expect to experience effects that last between 4 and 10 hours. These include dizziness, significant increase in one's confidence and motion of regular forms.

A small portion of the species that are representative from the Psilocybe class is:

Psilocybe cubensis.

The species is said to be the most famous of the Psilocybes. It is called cubes or shrooms. The species is found all over the globe. It's produced with the help of dairy animal fertilizers from The United States, Gulf of Mexico, Central America, South America, West Indies, Thailand, Cambodia, India and Australia.

They are easily identified by their conic-to-angled tops that can grow from 2 to 8 cm in size. The dark, reddish-cinnamon hue turns golden with time and also inspired the name of their road, gold tops.

It has psilocin in addition to psilocin and baeocystin. Due to the presence of certain components, such as the amount of all substances within this species vary.

Psilocybe Cyescens.

The type is also referred to as wavy tops, as a result of their tops , which get particularly wavy as they are formed. They are distinctive among their class due to its light yellowish and buffy hue.

The spores, which are dark and blackish-colored, are also distinct.

Within the United States, P. Cyanescens thrives within The Pacific Northwest, South of the San Francisco Bay zone. It also thrives throughout Western as well as Central Europe, Australia, West Asia, Western Europe, Central Europe, and New Zealand.

They are cultivated on woodchips that line the borders of urban zones as well as mulched beds. Due to the requirements for fruiting for this plant, cultivating them indoors is a challenge.

Psilocybe semilanceata.

The organism is found in fields, and is particularly prevalent in wet environments. Contrary to P. cubensis it doesn't grow from the waste of. It feeds on rotting grass and can be found in 17 countries within the Northern Hemisphere, particularly in North America, Canada, Russia, Switzerland, Poland as well as the Netherlands.

Semilanceatas are called freedom tops. Their tops range from 5 to 25mm in length, and change as they go from being channel-molded, to ring-shaped with a distinct top that resembles an.

Psilocybe azurescens.

This is the most potent psilocybin-containing mushrooms with psilocybin levels of 1.78%. Anyone who is who are new to magic mushrooms should not eat anything over one-eighth of P. Azurescens. It is extremely powerful and twice as strong than P. cubensis.

Psilocybe samuiensis

Magic mushrooms of this kind is found in rice paddies of Thailand especially located in Ranong Province, and is often referred to as hed Keequai. P. samuiensis' top is rhomboid with 7-15mm width, and it develops an intense red-dark-colored hue when moist. It's a small, unnoticeable change that is not more than 2 inches tall, and isn't particularly evident. The assets of this species are comparable to the larger P. cubensis.

Psilocybe Cyofibrillosa

A seashore creature of type, P. cyanofibrillosa are essential to flood fields and waterway estuaries that span across Northern California and British Columbia. They live in soils filled with wood debris. Tops vary in width between 1.4-3.5cm and are level as they the passage of time. The dark chestnut color changes from obscured spots change to a yellowish dark color or grayish-white after drying. "Rhododendron Psilocybe" and "Blue-Haired Psilocybe" are their names of origin and are believed for having effects that are slightly less powerful than P. cubensis.

Psilocybe mexicana

Like its name implies, as the name suggests. Mexicana is found in Mexico and other parts of Central America. Aztecs as well as Mayans have been using for a long time in a variety of capacities. They have been referring to them as "teonancatl" meaning "god's material."

Its top is thin measuring between 0.5-2cm across and has an elongated channel. The darker-colored top could appear beige-hued to straw-hued, and can be a bit blue when it is damaged. It is probably the least noticeable impact and is an exceptional variation, even though it is a tough psychonaut.

Psilocybe pelliculosa

P. P. pelliculosa is found in groups in the humus, timberland flotsam, jetsam as well as on greenery within coniferous forests within the Pacific Northwest area of North America. It's also abundantly distributed throughout British Columbia, Canada. It's often referred to as "Conifer Psilocybe"" because of its cone-molded top. As it matures it's top appears to be a complete chime mold and grows to around 0.8-2cm in the width. In terms of the power of the chime and how strong it is, it's considered to be an example of the "generally more delicate" kind of.

Psilocybe weilii

This living creature can be found from May until December. It can be located in soil that is red and that is dotted with pine needles. It is located in the north of Georgia, USA. The distinctive features of this plant are its taste and scent that resembles cucumber. P. weilii is also known for its white scale-like residues on its top. These can range from 3 to 6 centimeters in size. Although it's among the most rare psilocybin fungi, it's also believed to offer an experience that is shorter and less real.

Psilocybe Cyescens

The wavy top is a sure sign for P. cyanescens. Despite being called "Wavy-Capped Psilocybe." It's also known as "Cyan" as well as "Blue Halo." The species is increasing in the fall and winter throughout northern Pacific Northwest and is extensively distributed throughout all of the United Kingdom. However, the consumption of psilocybin is, by all accounts, greater within North American than Europe. Due to its efficacy it is highly sought-after by consumers across America. United States.

Psilocybe azurescens

Commonly referred to as commonly referred to as the Flying Saucer, Blue Runner, Blue Angel, Indigo Psilocybe and Astoriensis, this species grows throughout northwestern Oregon Coast near Astoria, Oregon. It is a fan of rise grasses and is a species that can be used in a variety of ways. Its top is 30 to 100mm, it is arched and conic. It grows to a point as it gets older. It's probably the most solid combination of mushrooms. One eighth of this mushroom could get rid of the problem within 30 minutes, and cause severe "migraines" the following day.

Psilocybe hispanica

According to the name, this species is located in Spain with a height over 2,300 meters. Spanish young people eat it due to its ability to alter minds, and evidence of the use of it in rituals that date back to 6000 years before. They are extremely resistant to freezing temperatures.

Psilocybe baeocystis

It was discovered on the rotting of conifer mulch It's typical of the species that is found in the Pacific, Northwest of the United States. They are often referred to as "Baeos" and "Bumpy Tops." The top edge turns into the inside of the body when you are young. Alongside the normal affects of psychoactivity, the ring also shows physical effects, such as the debilitated breathing, flushing of the skin.

Psilocybe Sylvatica

The species is cultivated from wood chips during the autumn. The sightings have been documented throughout Northern Europe, Eastern United States as well as Ontario, Canada. It's identified with p. that is pelliculosa. It can be identified by the condition on its highest.

Psilocybe stuntzii

Also known as "Stuntz's Blue Legs" This is another species of mushroom found within the Pacific Northwest of the United States. It blooms in late July and continues to grow until December. Despite its psychoactive properties It is best not to use this variety due to the nature it is physically similar to the dangerous G. marginata.

Amanita muscaria

The species isn't a source of the chemical psilocybin. The psychoactive effects of this species originate from the muscimol. A. Muscaria, also known as The Fly Agaric mushroom is beautiful with white pieces. It's pretty much the same as the shrooms in Alice in Wonderland, Super Mario Brothers and Fantasia. This one is particularly recommended for psychonauts who are in the frontline. A lot of first-time users report experiences that cause ailment as well as extreme sweating as the first effects. The beneficial effects are usually obtained after taking the drug twice or more times.The outcomes of the magic mushroom could be amazing, terrifying, or even completely absent. If you are aware of the various types that are available, you will be able to pick the one that best meets your psychedelic desires.

The cap is 30 to 100 millimeters in diameter. It straightens as you get older. They're found in coastal dunes grasses that cover a small portion that is located on the United States' West Coast. Germany is also home to some wild species.

Conocybe mushrooms

The majority of conocybe species are thin, long stems, with delicate leaves. They are found in lush grasslands, dead grass, dead greenery and the sand dunes, decayed wood and other the remains of. Conocybe species are referred to as cone heads due to their bell-shaped or conical caps.

The conocybe species contains at least 243 species of mushroom four of which contain the psychedelic compounds psilocin , and the psilocybin.

Conocybe kehneriana. It isn't much known about this fungus, however it is found throughout Norway as well as Argentina. Its appearance is similar to the usual highlights of who are part of Conocybe. Conocybe type.

Conocybe siligineoides.

Also known as cone beat its growth is delicate, small and only 3 inches tall. The top of the cone is a ringer with an orange-red tint. When spores begin to form the ringer, it develops an corroded shade.

It's not found in any areas of the world. The majority of examples were collected in Mexico which was the first place it was designated as a consecrated fungus utilized in various recuperation and healing ceremonies. They are consumed by the local population whether fresh or in tea.

Conocybe cyanopus/Pholiotina cyanopus.

The parasite was initially assigned as a member of the class Pholiotina however it was relegated to the Conocybe group in 1935. It's a tiny mushroom that develops on rotting matter , with a conic or the top which is a remarkably curly top. has a smooth, toned more dark.

It's basically little, typically less than 25mm in diameter and with stripes on the edges. The stem is soft and smooth with whitish areas at the bottom and tanish towards the top. The spores of this species are cinnamon-colored. Mycologists generally discourage the collection and consumption of this species due to the close resemblance with toxic species.

Another feature that this species has is the capacity to form sclerotias, which is a lazy form of the fruiting body that grows underground. Sclerotia are often referred to as truffles.

The species is found in fields, gardens, and in verdant areas in the areas with mild temperatures in North America, Austria, Belgium, Denmark, Finland, France, Germany, Germany, Hungary, Latvia as well as Latvia, the Netherlands,

Norway, Poland, Russia, Sweden, Switzerland, Ukraine, and the United States.

Conocybe Smithii/Pholiotina smithii. Similar to the species mentioned over, the species is currently being changing its name to the Pholiotina kind.

The P. Smithii can be located in North America, and much often, it grows in channels, marshes and swampy areas, mostly in sphagnum-colored greenery. It can also be seen along waterway banks as well as in yards. It's known to be found within Canada, Oregon, Wisconsin, Washington, and on the old earthen hills that were created by humans located in Northern Michigan. It is a natural product producer during the springtime.

Smithii's tops measure 0.3-1cm wide, with the shape of a conic or arched that grows to nearly the same height with time. The cinnamon-darker color of its concealing is consistent due to the color that its spores.

In spite of their subtle hallucinogenic effects strongly advise against using them in hallucinogenic tests due to the resemblance to dangerous mushrooms.

Copelandia/Panaeolus mushrooms

Copelandia is a family comprised of 12 species of fungi which are all thought as having stimulants such as Psilocin, and psilocybin. American as well as European mycologists have agreed to place mushrooms belonging to the Copelandia kind under Panaeolus.

Mushrooms from the Panaeolus family range from light from dark to tan with thin, long stems. They are found in the tropics and neotropics on opposite sides of equator. They are appearing in meadows, dead grass, dead greenery and sand rises, decayed wood and Fecal matter. Due to their psilocin-rich content they can be get injured and then turn blue.

Principal species of the Panaeolus class include:

Panaeolus cambodginiensis.

It is a powerful stimulant mushroom, which contains psilocybin as well as Psilocin. The top of the mushroom is less than 23mm in height, with an arched design. The top is smooth and has dim and dull looking gills. It's not surprising considering the spores that are too dim.

It thrives on the fertilizer of wild ox in water. It was first observed in Cambodia however it was discovered to be an array of categories across the Asian subtropics as well as Hawaii.

Panaeolus cyanescens.

Another psilocybin fungus that shares a space alongside the type previously mentioned. This one's peak is 1.5-4cm wide and it has an incurved edge as it grows. Its color ranges from gold to yellowish. However, it can turn blue or green when it is injured. The spores of the fungus are dark and stream-colored.

It's also a source of waste, with kinds that are found in pastures across Africa, Australia, parts of Asia, North America, and South America.

Panaeolus bisporus.

Physically the species doesn't seem to be distinct to the P. cambodginiensis. It could be isolated by an amplifier.

This tiny, darker-colored mushroom is grown on fertilizer and is covered in dull spores. It is located within Hawaii, Southern California, North Africa, Spain, and Switzerland.

Panaeolus tropicalis.

It is among the most powerful psilocybin mushroom in the Copelandia/Panaeolus species. The top is brown-shaded, 1.5-2.5cm wide, and is hemispheric or curving. The stem measures 5-12cm and then turns black at the point of the root. It turns blue after being injured.

Tropicalis also grows on fertilizers and is commonly located on the islands of Hawaii, Central Africa, and Cambodia. It is also expanding across Mexico, Tanzania, the Philippines, Florida, and Japan.

Galerina mushrooms

Galerina is a species of tiny, dark-colored spored mushrooms kind that grow on decaying matter, with more than 300 species around the globe, from the extreme north to the remote Macquarie Island in the Southern Ocean. Some species belonging to this classification are typically small and have a thin, delicate stem. They thrive on wood and overgrown habitats.

Of the many varieties of mushrooms belonging to the Galerina type There is one that is believed to release Psilocybin. The majority of the species are highly toxic.

Galerina steglichii.

It is a rarity in the world of magical mushrooms. They're only found once in Germany. They can be found in small numbers.

They can be identified by their dark-colored caps that are about 2mm in width. Their spores corrode to the shade of orange dull.

Inocybe mushrooms

Inocybe is a type made up of mushrooms-forming organisms. Populations of Inocybe are found within the host plants that have vascular structures. When you look at this from a different perspective Inocybe is among the most adaptable varieties of mushrooms.

Common mushrooms of this group are darker, regardless of the fact that some types are the lilac variety. Their tops are typically tiny and cone-shaped, however growing longer as they get older. Certain tops have a distinct smellthat is described as smelly or spermatic.

The four species in this family have been well-known for stimulating effects.

Inocybe aeruginascens.

The first case of this species was reported on June 15th in 1965. It is found in warm regions and have been observed in sandy soils with a damp, moist environment across Central Europe along with the western part of North America.

The mushrooms are small, with a an elongated top that is conic that is usually less than 5 centimeters in size. The top shading changes from light yellow to buff dark in color, typically with greenish stains, which disappear as the mushrooms dry. These spores have a smooth surface and have the structure of an earth's darker pattern.

They have psychoactive compounds baeocystin and psilocin in addition to a brand new substance that is referred to as the aeruginascin. As of now, aeruginescens is the most common kind of magic mushroom that can produces the aeruginascin.

Inocybe coelestium.

Magic mushrooms of this kind is widespread throughout Europe. The name "coelestium" is a reference to "celestials," the occupants of Mount Olympus. This is due to the hallucinogenic qualities of coelestium.

The physical characteristics are as common to all species of the Inocybe type.

Inocybe haemacta.

This species shares a striking likeness to I. Aeruginescens. The magical mushroom is found in the shoreline regions throughout Europe.

Inocybe tricolor.

This microorganism belonging to the Inocybe type is found in soft timberlands. It also contains the psilocin and Psilocin. It's located within Norway in central Europe. The top is a square dark to red and lighter toward the edges. It's generally 4cm wide. It produces spores that are in the ochre-tan to dark-tan color.

Mycena mushrooms

The huge variety is made of fungi that also thrive upon decaying matter. They measure over two centimeters across and can be identified by an spore print that is white and a tiny bell-shaped top and a delicate stem. The majority of mushrooms in Mycena are dull or dark.

They can be difficult to distinguish from other kinds of mushrooms and should be viewed under an some sort of amplifying device to distinguish. Certain groups are edible while others are poisonous. One group contains the drug psilocybin.

Mycena cyanorrhiza.

It's a tiny, white mushroom with a blue-colored base. It grows in forests on the wood, and it leaves the spores are white.

It is a potent psilocybin-based substance, however it's likely to be a fake positive. Its edibility claims to be proved wrong and it does not have a proof of use for hallucinogenic purposes.

Pluteus mushrooms.

The variety includes over 300 different species that live on wood or remains of wood. These species leave pink-colored spore prints, and Gills that do not belong to the stem.

Some of these are beautiful, however the majority of people consider their flavor in consistency and taste as average. A few of the mushrooms that belong to this category will be blue when injured this is a sign that they are psilocybin-rich.

Pluteus brunneidiscus.

Brunneidiscus is an Agric organism that was first discovered within Spain as well as the United States. It is found only on the wood of trees that have large leaves between June and November.

Pluteus salicinus.

This European hallucinogenic fungus grows on wood. It is easily identified through its silver-dim tops that vary between 2 and 8cm in length. There are also small scales near the center that are darker near the edge and appears to be transparent when it is wet. The stem is about 3-5cm long and is slightly swollen near the bottom.

A convergence between psilocybin as well as Psilocin in the dried test from P. salicinus is revealed in the range of 0.21-0.35 percent in addition to 0.011 and 0.05 percentages separately.

There are a variety of enchantment mushroom to meet all tastes. If you're looking to embark for a trip to the hallucinogenic realm it is possible to purchase online for enchantment truffles and choose from the many varieties of enchantment truffles that are available!

The reason we grow mushrooms

Growing mushrooms at home can be an enjoyable and potentially lucrative hobby. It's not hard to set up an environment that will provide mushrooms sprouts with the right conditions and nutrients essential to yield a large amount of mushroom. You can cultivate both shiitake and familiar mushrooms at your home. Each type of mushroom has distinct requirements for growth.

Light

Mushrooms can't extract nutrients from the sun like plants can, therefore they don't require light. However, they do not require a dark environment for growth. The best position to develop mushrooms in darkness is that the darkness helps preserve the humidity that mushrooms need to reproduce. A storm cellar provides ideal conditions for the cultivation of buttons of all kinds, including regular ones and the logs that are used to grow Shiitake mushrooms must be kept away from the direct light of the sun.

Moisture

Like other fungi, thrive best in humid environments. Common mushrooms require a moist growth dampness levels of 35-45 percent which is why they require soaking for up to 48 hours after the logs begin to dry. The ideal shiitake growing log must have dry bark as well as moist inside surfaces.

Temperature

They can grow at temperatures ranging from between 40 and 90 F. Shiitake logs should be kept in a secluded outdoor space or beneath trees to maintain their moisture and keep the ideal temperature. Fans or heaters could be crucial to achieve the controlled conditions that mushroom species that require inside.

Nutrients

The essential nutrients mushrooms require in order to develop include sugar, starchand lignin and protein, as well as fats and nitrogen. Fertilizers made of straw and compost has the ideal quantities of these nutrients to grow common mushrooms while shiitakes can get the nutrients they require by consuming the wood from sawdust or wood that they are growing. A mix of peat moss, corn and sand can be an alternative to straw and compost.

Mushrooms are rich in fiber and vitamins. They're extremely adaptable and an excellent sources of protein and nutrients for those who are vegetarian. With all the varieties of mushroom, your options are endless.

Chapter 4: Listing Of The Most Commonly Used

Types Of Mushrooms

1. White Common Mushroom

Eatable mushroom referred to as Agarius Bisporuswhich has two different shade states when it is immature: brown and white, each with distinct names. If it is mature, it's commonly referred to as portobello.

White button mushrooms are the young and white variety. A mixture of peat moss, corn and sand provides an alternative to straw and compost.

They are rich in fiber and vitamins. They're adaptable and are an excellent sources of protein and nutrients for those who are vegetarians. With the variety of mushrooms to choose from, the possibilities are endless.

Cooked or raw, it can be used in stews, soups, pizzas, salads, and stews.

2. Crimini mushroom

Also known as: when it is young and dark-colored Agaricus bisporus is also known by the name of Cremino mushroom. Swiss brown mushrooms, Roman mushrooms, brown Italian darker

Most of the time, Criminis are portobello that is in its early stages and is sold as baby portobello, and they are basically ordinary white mushrooms that are not fully developed. White button and Crimini mushrooms can be interchanged. They're similar to fiddles, however they are slightly larger in size, and more dark in shade The crimini are an ethereal shade of dark-colored.

3. Portobello mushroom

Also known as field mushroom, also known as open-top shroom.

Additionally, if you require substitute for bread buns then you can make use of the flat top of the mushroom. They're ideal to grill and stuff.

4. Shiitake mushroom

Also known as Shitake Dark Timberland, dark oak, black winter, Chinese black, black mushroom

Oriental black, forest mushrooms Brilliant oak Donko.

Shiitake are a type of mushroom that grows predominantly throughout Japan, China, and Korea that is one of the main reasons they are so common within Asian food. In Japanese the word shiitake is a reference to "oak fungus," however, nowadays, the majority of cultivating shiitakes is done. They are characterized by a slight smell and woodsy scent as well as dried counterparts that are more pronounced.

5. Clam mushroom

Also known as: Pleurotus, tree shellfish, holy messenger's wings, pleurotte en huitre, abalone mushroom.

Clam mushrooms are a species of Pleurotus and are discovered in nature, thriving in the midst of trees. Nowadays, they're the most frequently grown edible mushrooms in the world. The trumpet of the ruler is the most renowned species of the type of shellfish mushrooms.

They're nutritious to cook and provide an extremely sweet and delicate season. They are typically used in saute or pan-fried meal because they're small and cook more evenly as compared to other mushrooms.

6. Enoki mushroom

Also known as Enokitake, enokidake, futu mushroom, winter mushrooms the winter growth or lily.

Enoki mushrooms can be purchased fresh or in canned form. The experts recommend eating fresh enoki that have crisp, white, and shiny tops. This is in contrast to ones with a sour or natural stalks which are better avoided. They're delicious unrefined and are a must in Asian cooking. Because the freshness of them, they stand up well in soups, and they work well with mixed greens. You can also utilize them in various recipes.

7. Chanterelle mushroom

Additionally, it is known as Golden yellow, chanterelle eggs, Girolle the pfifferling

Chanterelles are one of the most distinctive types of mushrooms found in the wild. They're yellow, orange or white, big and trumpet-shaped. Because they are difficult to cultivate and are difficult to find, chanterelles are often sought by nature. They're popular in a variety of European cuisines, such as French and Austrian and are similarly popular across America. United States.

Certain varieties possess a fruity scent and others have a more unpleasant, woody scent while others could be considered to be spicy. They are delicate with flavor and texture, and can be when sauteed or singed in margarine or oil or cream. They can be used as a starter smudge on bruschetta, or even mix the eggs with them. They are equally good in cream sauces, souffles soups, pasta, or souffles.

They are dark trumpets also known as dull the chanterelle, the Horn of Abundance, or the trumpet from the deceased. Dark trumpets possess a rich smokey flavor and scents of a truffle that is dark when dried.

8. Porcini mushroom

Also called: Porcino mushroom, Cepe bolete, Bolete, Ruler bolete, Borowik Polish mushrooms,

Steinpilz and stensopp. Also known as penny bun, or penny.

A big mushroom, similar to the portobello and the porcini, they are both mushrooms that are commonly utilized to make Italian cooking. Its taste has been described as slightly sweet and nutty with smooth, rich surfaces with a distinct aroma that is reminiscent of the sourdough. Fresh porcinis aren't so easily available within the United States. However, dried ones can be easily reconstituted by placing them in hot water for about 15 minutes before cooking. They're fantastic sauteed in margarine, then ground into pasta, used in soups, risottos, or in a myriad of meals. They're also among the only two mushrooms species that are salted and available economically.

9. Shimeji Mushroom

Also known as: Many species are sold under the name shimeji mushrooms such as buna-shimeji and bunapi-shimeji.

Shimeji is best cooked. It's not an excellent food item to serve raw due to its unpleasant flavor. The sharpness of the mushroom disappears completely when it is cooked, and the mushrooms become slightly sweet and nutty. This is one of the mushrooms that are delicious in cooking: sauteed meals and stews, in soups and stews and in a broad assortment of sauces.

10. Morel Mushroom is also known as morchella.

Of the different types of mushrooms These distinct microorganisms possess the appearance of honeycombs at the top. Morels are adored by chefs who are gourmet, especially in French foodbecause they are beautiful and delicious. Because of the difficulties in expanding, the business social event of wild morels has transformed into a multimillion dollar industry in the tranquil Northern Hemisphere, explicitly in North America, Turkey, China and in the Himalayas, India, and Pakistan in which these highly sought-after growths are in large quantities.

The most effective and least difficult methods to enjoy morels is slowly sautéing them in margarine. Then, sprinkle them with spice and salt. They're chewy, but taste delicious. Serve them alongside meat and poultry, or mix them into soups or pasta fillings.

THE MUSHROOM LIFE THE CYCLE

The cycle of life of mushrooms is, to a large degree, inaccessible to mushroom trackers, but not to mushroom cultivators. The mushroom cultivator follows the pattern of the cycle of life of the mushroom. Fruitbodies develop precisely in line with the cycle of life of mushrooms and, in the majority of species, appear in a few days, and then disappear.

Vaccination:

Spores appear on a growth substrate (or the substrate). In the event that the conditions are favorable that they will be, spores will grow.

Spore germination:

Fine contagious filaments, also known as hyphae are formed from spores. Hyphae that have a perfect mate form mature mycelium.

Mycelial extension:

Mycelium growth separates natural issues and absorbs nutrients from its state. In this stage of development mycelium expands at an astounding rate. It faces numerous predators and rivals that it smothers with an amazing display of defensive proteins and mix. In this regard mycelium is the defense mechanism of the mushroom.

Hyphal hitch

Mycelium grows into hyphal ties that then transform the form of "primordia" or baby mushrooms.

Primordia method of action

The mushroom creates an amazing display of impetuses, and also improves the components of both the mycelium as well as the fruitbody, which is growing. Host Defense gathers its harvest during the apex stage of development, resulting in an endless array of constituents, which includes polysaccharides (beta-glucans and arabinoxylanes) triterpenoids, glycoproteins and ergosterols and myco-supplements.

Fruitbody option:

From the many primordia the living organism chooses the most encouraging ones to grow into fruit bodies.

Grow Fruitbody:

The organism channelizes the bulk of its energy as well as supplements to construct the body of the fruit and eventually produce spores. Spore age refers to the sexual phase of the life cycle.

Spore discharge:

The fruit body releases seeds into the environment to spread. They arrive on the perfect medium (or developing medium) will grow, thereby beginning the cycle of life!

Street names for Psilocybin

The majority of drug dealers do not sell psilocybin under its original name. Instead, the drug can be sold under the following name:

Dangers:

Psilocybin users who have used the drug in uncontrolled situations may be in contact with reckless conduct like driving drunk.

Certain people may experience frequent, disturbing changes in how they perceive the world. The effects are always visual and may last anywhere between weeks and years following taking the stimulant.

Doctors presently analyze this condition as Hallucinogen-persisting perception disorder (HPPD), generally called a flashback. Flashbacks are a repulsion recall of an extremely upsetting information. The vivid memory of this disturbing background in psychedelic use is a horrifying experience or a fantasy that turns into a gruelling nightmare.

Some people have more negative results than mind-flights like anxiety, confusion, fear or psychosis and scattered symptoms that are similar to schizophrenia, which requires a trip to an emergency room.

Additionally, a doctor will treat these contacts using medications, such as benzodiazepines. These symptoms usually subside within between 6 and 8 hours after their effects due to the drug are fading away.

The risk is minimal Some psilocybin users are at risk of accidental injury from eating poisonous mushrooms accidentally.

The symptoms of a mushroom ache could be muscle cramps, chaos and even insaneness. See an emergency room immediately in the event of these symptoms.

Because psychedelic and other poisonous mushrooms are found in the majority of living areas it is recommended that individuals remove any and all mushrooms from places that children frequent to avoid accidental use.Most accidental consumption of mushrooms can bring an indigestion that is not severe however, only the most severe cases needing medical intervention.

PSILOCYBIN ABSUSE POTENTIAL

Psilocybin does not cause addiction chemically and there are no physical signs when you stop using it.

But, regular use may make a person intolerant to the effects the psilocybin. The same can happen with other substances, such as LSD as well as mescaline. Users of these substances have to hold their breath in any case for a few days between doses in order to feel the full effects.

After a long period of psilocybin consumption, individuals may feel a sense of mental fatigue and experience difficulties adjusting to their surroundings.

Myths and COMMON QUESTIONS

There are a myriad of myths surrounding magic mushrooms. Many people believe the fact the fact that magical mushrooms can be "safer" and give an "milder" experience as compared to other hallucinogenics.

Additionally, some people develop tolerance to psilocybin pretty quickly, which makes it difficult to experience any effects over a long period of usage.

Despite their potential to cause harm to anyone who consumes them, magic mushrooms can be as unpredictable in their effects as other drugs. Certain people have made public statements of significantly more alarming and extreme mind-flashes with magical mushrooms than LSD.

Various people also confuse fly agaric mushrooms with psilocybin-containing mushrooms--yet they are not the same. The fly agaric mushroom contains Ibotenic, a psychoactive chemical synthetic as well as the muscimol that is well-known to cause sweating, drooling, jerking as well as retching, tipsiness and even madness.

TOLERANCE and DEPENDENCE.

Like all medicines in the long run, the more you utilize Magic mushrooms the greater resistance you will develop. Resistance increases quickly as you go through the normal use. This means you require more to achieve similar results. The process of building up resistance using shrooms can be particularly dangerous since consuming a large amount can cause overdose-related symptoms that, although not deadly could lead to the result of irritation, retching, loose muscles, insides and suspicion or frenzy seizures and psychosis.

How long will PSILOCYBIN CONTINUE TO REMAIN IN YOUR INTERNET SYSTEM?

The short-term effects of magic mushrooms usually disappear within 6 to 12 hours, however, customers may experience changes in personality and flashbacks after having consumed the pills.

The usual half-life of psilocybin can range from an hour to two and in the majority of cases will take between five and six hours for the substance to disappear from your body.

The standard pee medicine screening for business does not detect psilocybin. However there are tests which can be used to determine the significance of the drug. Like other drugs Magic mushrooms can be detected in hair follicles up to 90 days.

How long does Psilocybin stay in your system?

Habit

Psilocybin isn't addictive, and it doesn't cause a need for immediate usage. This is usually due to the basis that the medication can trigger a severe "trip."

WITHDRAWAL

While most users experience physical withdrawal symptoms as they stop taking the tranquilizer, some report psychological symptoms, which could include depression.

How to Find Help

If you suspect that your teenager is using or experimenting regularly with magical mushrooms, you should have a calm and gentle discussion with them regarding the dangers of psychedelics, particularly when mixed with other drugs or any kind of alcohol. If you suspect this, you must make sure that they know that you're available to offer all kinds of assistance and support.

A FEW TIPS FOR TAKING MUSHROOMS: A BEGINNER'S GUIDE

M

Aic mushrooms have been used over the years to provide memories that span from exhilarating to awe-inspiring. Anyhow, newbies should plan their trip with care and follow some guidelines to ensure that your initial and subsequent excursions are ones you'd like to recreate.

Consuming the magic Mushrooms provides an experience unlike any other. They've been around for centuries in various cultures to facilitate spiritual interactions and an experience of being connected to the Divine.

Like all medication that is psychoactive it is important to be mindful when taking the medication. According to Timothy Leary stated, "set and set" have plenty of tasks to accomplish.

You'll feel good once you begin running

Shrooms can boost moods and moods you're experiencing when you consume these. If you're struggling with depression or feeling unwell, depressed, there's the possibility that you'll have a negative experience.

Relax and be in a confident setting

You should be in a secure location and surrounded by people who whom you can know. A poor or "heavy" excursion in a difficult situation on your own or with strangers could result in an unpleasant experience. It is strongly recommended, especially for people who are truffle enthusiasts and mushroom novices, to take an "sitter" accompanying you throughout your entire journey. A"sitter" is someone who is calm, who ensures everything runs smoothly and makes sure that you and your companions traveling with you at relaxed.

Get yourself set up

Make sure you have water, organic drinks, tea leaves and a light bite made and ready. The effects that magic truffles produce are evident and shouldn't be overlooked. They are well-respected within 3-6 hours. but you might not be hungry. It might be difficult to locate the icebox. Therefore, make sure to have food available.

Enjoy magic truffles on an empty stomach.

However, avoid eating anything for at most three hours prior to taking the mushrooms. In this way the psilocybin can be taken in also.

What quantity of magical mushrooms should I take?

There isn't a "should" regarding dosage. It's best to stay slow and study one's conventional side. If you've never tried shrooms or are a truffle amateur, you probably do not realize that you're so sensitive to the psilocybin. If you're okay with it being sensitive, keep in mind that truffle measurements differ from those of mushrooms.

There are some examples you can use to judge. A quarter of one gram of dried shrooms can be described as to be the "edge parcel." It means that a person will experience a mild encounter and will not notice any effects. This is why you might notice that bright shades and intense lights acquire an "starry" appearance, but little more. The eyes might become wider and you might experience a mild discomfort or be faced with "mental journeys" that want to create curves around your vision's fringe.

A "medium" amount of 1-2.5gm is a great excursion. When feeling nausea. Eyes will grow, and your pulse may increase (in spite of it is not at an unhealthy degree). Different users get an "cooling" impression that grows more solid as the journey progresses. The signs that are visible appear just like the fantasies-like images of the shroom journeys. The feelings will also be intense and exaggerated. This is why it's important to have a trusted sitter especially for those who aren't experienced. The most frequent negative issues in this period are unusual self-questioning. The "sense of self-misfortune" similar to the way it is that users experience is often presented, in the proper situation, as an amazing experience, that means a complete fulfillment of one's situation, without the absence of any particular desire, difficulty or control.

Are magic mushrooms dangerous?

There isn't a definitive answer to this question, but in the end, the correct answer is not. There aren't any documented cases of fatal overdoses and psilocybin hasn't been deemed dangerous. Psilocybin mushrooms also won't make you forget reality. You won't be diagnosed with schizophrenia or have a psychotic episode, and your experience won't last forever. But in the event that you have an underlying psychological disorder and/or mental illness, it may aggravate those ailments. For the majority of us, mushrooms are the most safe hallucinogenic options available.

What's a good way to travel?

It is entirely dependent on the user. The hues of the articles become very distinct. Users will also feel joy, and laugh at the absurdity of things. There will be a resounding sound and you could be unsure if they were real in any way that you could imagination. You'll also be able to "see" amazing geometric examples that change into various forms when you shut your eyes. People who have this experience feel a sense of "opportunity" to think rationally. The lines of reasoning flow efficiently, and some shroom trippers have an "superior perception" of their lives. A few people also say they "converse with the heavens" or have "different perceptions" of cognition.

What are MUSHROOM SPORES?

The spores of mushrooms are small and regenerative cells that enable can be found in all living things to reproduce and expand. Spores are found in large quantities on healthy mushrooms due to their germination is only possible in unique circumstances. Each spore serves as an identification card for the kind of mushroom from which it originated which is a significant fact for those who track wild mushrooms and have to identify a variety to ensure safe use.

Definition

The mushroom spore an unicellular life form that is that is responsible for the conceptual structure of mushroom-making organisms. In his book "Eatable Mushrooms" Clyde Martin Christensen reports that the spores measure just 1/2500 inches long. Spores are located in the lower part of the on the top, inside the gills and teeth or the pores of the mushroom. Gills, teeth, as well as pores are the indication of the dimensions and shape of the spore-conveying location of the mushroom.

Conditions

Some mushrooms do not produce spores often. Mushrooms are similar to the things on a tree, and the seed is represented in the spores. Like natural trees, create green foods that can multiply provided there are enough nutrients and water to define the additional energy required to produce spores. So, the majority of mushrooms are a sign of a growing system which is healthy because they are copying.

Capacity

Spores drop or are sucked away from the top of the mushroom. Their tiny size permit them to be caught within, and then carried by delicate air flow. When the majority of spores land they land on the barren ground, such as leaves, rocks and streams. The spores that land on fertile ground release shoots that fall into the ground, and find various shoots, derived from different spores , and establishing the process of regenerative regeneration, working with in the development of the underground organisms' system.

Spore Prints

The distinction between wild and edible mushrooms is an important method to use because a wide variety of mushrooms can be poisonous, and eating them could cause serious health problems, at any time and at times. A spore print is just one of the techniques employed to identify different types of mushrooms. In order to make a spore image it is necessary to remove the top on the mushrooms is removed and placed gill-, teeth- or pore-side down on a white paper or Cling wrap. By placing a bowl on the top of the mushroom and allowing it to stay in the medium-term, it will trigger the mushroom to release numerous spores. After a whole day, the sum of spores radiated will be an impression, a unique that can be played with and shaded to distinguish the various types of the mushrooms.

Kinds of Wild Mushrooms

Chanterelle mushrooms are found in the wild all over the globe, and is generally known under the designation "splendid Chanterelle" within North America. The chanterelle is extensively utilized by experts in the field of gourmet because of its flavor and aroma and is among a handful of mushrooms that are consistent in its shading. If you want to cultivate the chanterelles from spores it is recommended to try it in the wild since there is no way to cultivate the mushroom locally beginning in 2011. If you decide to plant Chanterelles in the wild the conditions need to be perfect for an abundant harvest.

Things You'll require

* Chanterelle mushroom

* Soil analyzer

* Garden rake

Find a tree that provides the ideal conditions for chanterelle mushroom to develop. Achieving high yields from chanterelles is generally caused by trees due to the fact that they share positive relationships. The most exceptional trees are beech, cleanpine, Birch. The ideal environment for chanterelles to thrive is one with soil that drains well and is low in nitrogen.

Check the soil close to the tree. The ideal pH of the soil falls somewhere within the range of 4 to 5.5. The ideal soil for the growth of chanterelles, in the main part, is the one with the highest possible pH. However, if the soil in the area you'd like to develop isn't in the proper parity, you can increase levels by adding lime, or using sodium chloride to reduce the levels. If you notice several chanterelles in the area you'd like to expand There is a good likelihood that the soil is of the ideal pH.

Make sure you rake the dirt in the area on the spot where you would like to create the chanterelle spores as they will not survive in the soil that is bare. In the future, avoid walking around on the soil.

The chanterelle mushroom is broken up and placed on top of the soil you dug and then carefully scatter the pieces all over. Chanterelles produce small amounts of spores which are tiny, and aren't able to fit into an area. It is therefore perfect for spreading pieces of the fungus on soil as they hold the seeds inside them and on the. If you want to increase your chances of growing chanterelles might want to try with more than one.

Let the pieces of mushrooms that you spread out in peace. Chanterelles grow well on the soil they nature when the conditions are favorable.

Tips and Advice

The ideal time to grow Chanterelle mushrooms is during July.

It is ideal to utilize chanterelle mushrooms which haven't been cleaned. The washing of chanterelles can expel its spores.

When the chanterelle is left unaffected, it will continue to grow each year. Beware of planting seeds of chanterelle next to the tree with mycorrhizae fungi as it could cause competition and possibly kill the spores you've planted.

The mushrooms that grow in circles are known as fairy rings. Mushroom spores, also known as mycelium, can be found in a variety of soil kinds. They're even found in some soil mixes that haven't been sterilized with high temperatures. While the majority of mushroom spores never grow into a full-blown mushroom, periods of continuous rain and watering can create a mushroom appearance. Although they can be ugly however, they pose no danger to your garden and you can get rid of them by hand to prevent them from growing.

Things You'll Be Needing

Shovel

Garbage bag

Nitrogen fertilizer

Manure spreader

Water

Use a scoop that is four inches away from the mushroom and then dig down to 5 inches to lift this mushroom off the soil. Then, gently place the mushroom in the trash bag made of plastic so that it doesn't scatter seeds, which can cause the growth of new mushrooms. Repeat the process to dig into all remaining mushrooms.

Pour pure nitrogen fertilizer into the spreader for manure and set the spreader's dial to release at a rate of one Lb per 1000 square feet of lawn.

The lawn's overboard along with other lines to spread nitrogen fertilizer.

The garden should be watered lightly to saturate the nitrogen in the soil. Nitrogen helps soil break down organic matter faster and removes the main food source for mushrooms.

Tips and Warns

To prevent mushrooms from growing again To prevent the growth of mushrooms, get rid of all organic matter like pine straw, mulch as well as pet waste, from the garden. Also, take away dead stumps of trees or logs which are a source of food for mushrooms.

Avoid using fertilizers with slow release. It is essential for nitrogen to be released as fast as possible in order to eradicate the mushrooms.

Mushroom spawn is actually mycelium that has been created on different substances. Mycelium is a spore of mushrooms which have been grown. Mushroom spawn is utilized more than spores from mushrooms to produce mushrooms since the spores are not always reliable, however the spores germinated by the spores are only able to be stored for a certain period of time. When you purchase mushrooms spawn, it is best be planning to use all of it. If you do have an unopened jar, you may keep it in storage to extend the shelf life.

Things You'll require

* Mushroom generate

* Cooler

Keep track of the date on the cluster of mushrooms. The mushrooms that are delivered economically should have the date when the mycelium was incorporated into the substrate. Because they are living, they are also susceptible to microorganisms in shape, and the mesothelial waste that it produces.

Make sure you use all of your mushrooms supply after receiving it. The faster you begin using it the more mushrooms you'll harvest. The longer you keep it in your home, the more it degrades.

Store any mushrooms that are not being used in their original containers. Be careful not to transfer the mycelium to a different container. The original packaging it came with was designed specifically to store the mushroom delivery.

Keep the mushroom that is not used in a cooler that is customized to be somewhere between the range of 32 to temperatures of 35 degrees F. The mushroom's produce can be kept for two months.

Tips and Advice

* Utilize all of your mushrooms as fast as you can prior to the mycelium begins to die.

References

* Penn State College of Agricultural Sciences and Six Steps to Mushroom Farming; Daniel J. Royse, and others.

* Mushroom-Appreciation.com: Grow Mushrooms with Mushroom Spawn* To what extent Can You Keep Fresh Mushrooms in the Refrigerator?

* The most effective way to ensure that mushrooms are kept fresh

* What Are Mushroom Spores?

* Many kinds of wild mushrooms thrive in Oregon.

Oregon offers a assortment of mushrooms native to the state. Some are edible while some are poisonous. They are usually akin to edible species. It is often difficult to differentiate the different types when you find wild mushrooms. It is best to avoid eating these types of mushrooms when you are certain that they're safe.

Moreels

Morels are one of the most popular kinds of mushrooms found in Oregon and are consumed and is a consumable mushrooms grows in the spring, and is often located on mountains. They have a distinct heading , which is located in the top portion of the plant as well as at the top of the stal. they are much easier to spot compared to other wild mushrooms.

Kingh Bolete

Kingh Bolete or more popularly known as Boletus Edulis is a species that is found throughout the forests in the Pacific Northwest. It is characterized by a brown or yellow cap, and an elongated white-to-brown stalk. The bolete that is the ruler is harvested in the fall and is sold at claim to famed restaurants and nourishment markets.

White Matsutake

The white matsutake is a common plant in the state's favorable climate and is often located in mixed coniferous woodlands. It is located in both the waterfront and the inland forests of this state, and is harvested between November and December. It is often found in close proximity to plants as rhododendron, huckleberry and r in accordance with the U.S. Forest Service.

Chantarelle

The chantarelle mushroom can be located in a variety of zones in The Pacific Northwest, including Oregon's Willamette National Forest. It's most common within Douglas forest, a type of fir but it may be found close to the live oak tree. It has a yellow-orange top and a white underneath that is harvested during autumn or winter. It is also harvested in spring. Its spring crop is dependent on cold weather, states the U.S. Timberland Service.

How do you identify EDIBLE FUNGUS AND MUSHROOMS

How to identify Mushrooms

For example, Ohio is home to over 2,000 varieties of wild mushrooms as according to The Ohio State University. While some of them are edible, there are others that are dangerous and it's unclear whether it is protected to consume the majority of the species. Mushrooms are a part of scenes in Ohio which is awash with them for any mushroom hunter to be content.

Chanterelle

The most sought-after edible mushrooms that grows within Ohio is the chanterelle. It is also known as Cantharellus Cibarius. this medium-sized fungus is green or yellow depending on the shading. Chanterelles do not have gills similar to other types of mushrooms, but they do have has edges and overlays on the top. According to the Ohio State University, they usually grow from June through September, in an oak tree's shade. Trackers with tenderfoots must be cautious when collecting chanterelles, especially since they resemble the poisonous jack-o'-lamp mushroom.

Mammoth Puffball

Mammoth Puffballs are an undisputed mushroom that is found in Ohio. Sometimes referred to as Calvatia gigantea These goliaths are very tasty and are generally seen in late August to October.

The goliath-shaped puffball, that is usually white, is named due to its appearance. It is A massive white ball that could grow in widths of between eight and 24 inches, allowing that of Ohio State University. Monster puffballs prefer to grow in open areas, such as for instance, in parks, mountains and pastures, as well as in urban areas.

Destroying Angels

The the destroying angel is a deadly mushroom that has been found in Ohio. Similar to the Amanita bisporigera The destroying angel is characterized by long white shafts that have a smooth, balanced top. They are typically seen between July and October, and are found in forest areas. According to The Cornell Mushroom Blog the destroying angel can harm the liver, and a significant percentage of those who consume the destroying angel suffer. If you happen to consume a destroying angel and you are unable to identify it, call an immediate toxin control and visit a specialist.

There are a variety of methods for salvaging mushrooms. Mushrooms are protected to extend their shelf life. The fresh mushrooms are stored for five days or more after picking. The mushrooms that are protected can be stored for a longer period of time (even up to 5 years!)

The shielding industry shapes fresh mushrooms in a variety of ways. After the mushrooms are picked on the farm, they are transported to the processing plants at the speed that is sensible in context of the present situation. The mushrooms are immediately placed in a vacuum, where they take in a significant amount of water. They are a great source of air. When they are placed in a vacuum, they are replaced by water, which means they will not float onto the surface in the pot that brightens.

The process of whitening mushrooms (dip them into the boiling liquid) is the beginning phase to increase the duration of useability. Through warming, the mushrooms are less susceptible to becoming weak. The mushrooms travel along a conveyor belt and are cut by a machine and then the ice water cools them then they are dried and then they are tucked away out of the belt into massive plastic containers or buckets. The only thing required is an hour to turn 10 kilograms of fresh mushrooms into a bag. Once they are cool, they will stay for around one month and a half.

In the final step that mushrooms are cleaned or sanitized to ensure they remain in all circumstances to be sanitized and cleansed. Purification is when the mushrooms are heated to temperatures of 95 degrees Celsius for a period of time which extends the shelf lifespan to about a half an entire year (as that the mushrooms remain in a refrigerated area). In the event of the need for cleansing then the mushrooms are heated up to the temperature of 125 degrees Celsius. The purified containers can be kept up to a maximum to five years.

Storing mushrooms in oil, vinegar or salt

They can also be kept in oil or vinegar. The majority of Eastern Europe they, for the majority of time, utilize vinegar. However, storage with oil is commonplace across the Mediterranean. One notable example is mushrooms in the form of food items as an Italian appetizer or a starter. In China mushrooms are typically kept in salt. The separations for securing the production line in

China are huge and make it difficult to clean fresh mushrooms. The disadvantage of storing them within salts is that they have to be rinsed with a massive amount of water to prevent the taste from being excessively salty. This does not improve the taste. That's one reason people from all over the world choose Dutch secured mushrooms. Since the handling industry and the growers are within close proximity and the mushrooms can be harvested quickly after harvesting. This is why Dutch mushrooms have a healthy fresh season regardless of whether they are the mushrooms are pressed into a can or container, a pack or bucket.

How to Store FRESH MUSHROOMS

* Tips for Capacity

* Freezing

* Drying

* Utilizing

If you properly store fresh mushrooms they'll last for up to one week. It's simple. Here's how.

Place your entire, unwashed, mushrooms in a dark-colored bag. Fold the top of the bag over. Then, you can place the bag inside the primary section of your fridge. The pack is able to absorb any dampness that comes of the mushrooms ensuring that they don't become damp or spongy.

Tips for storing your mushrooms

Don't store mushrooms in your vegetable cabinet because it's too humid and sloppy.

Avoid placing them near food items with strong aromas or tastes since they'll absorb them like sponges.

A variety of well-known mushrooms can be kept more effectively in coolers as compared to other species. To reduce waste, you should make sure you buy your mushrooms prior to the time you intend to make use of them.

If you must keep mushrooms in storage for more than 7 days, you should think about drying or forming them into a solid.

How to Freeze Mushrooms

They are a great freezer, but it's best to place them into the cooler as quickly as they are available. Be sure to not delay your harvest, so the mushrooms don't begin to fall apart in the ice box before you set up some aside. If you've got a big mushrooms, you should focus on preparing some to consume and others to eat later. Make sure you are realistic regarding the amount you'll consume over the next week, so you can store the rest before they get rotten.

Mushrooms must be cooked prior to when they are frozen. This will prevent the chemical activity in this manner, and will preserve their quality. It's crucial to not skip this step.

Step-by-step instructions on how to dry Mushrooms

If your home doesn't offer plenty of cool space to dedicate to mushrooms drying them out is an alternative option. The dried mushroom can be used to rehydrate if needed, and take up little space. Make use of a low-temp oven or a dehydrator that can nourishment for drying your mushroom. Keep them in a tightly sealed holder until you're ready to use them.

If you've never dried mushrooms before, try a tiny amount to observe your thoughts. If you can figure out how you can reconstitute them, you might discover that they retain their original shape. In any case, it's wonderful that you have dried mushrooms in your pantry to use in homemade soups.

The most effective way to freeze mushrooms the right Way

* Frozen mushrooms

Clean and prep

* Make a meal Before Freezing

* Fast Freeze

The most efficient method to utilize Mushrooms

There are many ways to preserve them.

If you're a fan of mushrooms then you'll want to stock up on your favorite varieties of mushrooms during the time of season and small. You can then store them until you're ready to use them in all of your favorite recipes.

Choose mushrooms that appear like they are fresh and smell good. The mushrooms that look dry or shriveled, covered in a dark haze or spoiled, with a number of terrible spots or have a sour smell should be avoided. Choose only those that's in good condition.

Strategies to use up mushrooms

If you're not in a position to control your mushrooms before they turn bad, here are couple of ideas. Include them in pasta dishes or use them to make a topping for pizza or add them to soups or sauté them in spreads and then add them to hamburgers. Sauteed mushrooms can also be delicious as a side dish to steak. Just flip through your recipe gatheringand you'll be sure to come across a myriad of recipes that taste fantastic with a lot of mushrooms sprinkled in.

Clean your mushrooms with warm water, then trim the ends that are not bargains. Any mushrooms larger than 1 inch in across should be cut in quarters or cut into pieces.

The effects of freezing can alter the shade and appearance of mushrooms, rendering them more dark and soft.

Steamed mushrooms live a more prolonged and dragged out time than sauteed or steamed mushrooms.

Making a meal for freezing

Mushrooms must be cooked prior to freezing. There are two methods to accomplish this:

Sauteeing:

The mushrooms should be cooked in a skillet that has been browned using a tiny amount of oil or butter over high temperature. They should cook for approximately five minutes and until they're completely cooked and a significant part of the liquid disappears.

Chapter 5: Mycology: Growing Magic Mushroom

The majority of mushroom farmers begin with Psilocybin cubensis. It is the most well-known and easy to grow. There are many methods of making mushrooms, but we'll concentrate on the one that's the easiest. A spore can be the primary starting point for all methods. One spore can develop into a single fungus, which could produce hundreds of thousand spores.

The prints of Spores are utilized to cultivate mushrooms and can also be used to determine the species of wild mushrooms. To use them the dry spores that appear printed on the image must be humidified. In every aspect of cultivating, sterilization is crucial as mold or bacteria can stop them from growing even if they do, but this could also result in poisonous mushrooms. Instead of making your own, many growers purchase the syringes for spores (loaded with spores, the sterile water) from suppliers.

A big glass container made of plastic, canned jars canner or pressure cooker and brown rice flour vermiculite (a mineral-based gravel that is used to create potting plant) and other kitchen appliances are among other things you need. The brown rice flour gets mixed with vermiculite and water in order to create a soft, loose cake of substrate that creates the perfect environment for mushrooms to grow. spores to grow. The substrate is put into canning jars. They will be sterilized, sealed and sealed inside the pressure cooker or in a canner.

The surface is infected by the spore syringe that has been that are drilled into the lids of the jars once the jars have been cooled. The spores are then incubated at an average temperature of 75°F for a number of hours (23.9 temperatures Celsius). Within a week, spores are expected to begin to form and look like white fluff ropes, also called mycelium. If the mold develops in place of the bacteria there is no growth it is likely that something has gone wrong. It could be that you didn't sterilize your equipment sufficiently or introduced contaminants into the process of inoculation.

The cakes are then placed inside the plastic container to begin fruiting after they are coated with mycelium. The cakes are subjected to sunlight and plenty of humidity in the container. After a few weeks the mushrooms will begin to grow and be ready for picking when caps begin tilting upwards. Every cake could yield mushrooms for at least a month through what's known as flushes. These are formed in waves. A single cake of mushrooms can produce a plethora of mushrooms. Because they decay rapidly and are often stored in a refrigerator or dried to ensure they are fresh.

A few enthusiastic growers move from these simple methods to methods for bulk-growing. The bulk growing substrate could include things like manure or straw that needs to be pasteurized to avoid the growth of mold. When executed correctly, could produce thousands or hundreds of mushrooms in one harvest.

The cost of growing mushrooms isn't prohibitive however, getting the spore prints or syringes for spores can be difficult because purchasing, sellingor even having mushrooms isn't usually allowed.

This guide is inspired by Robert McPherson's "Psylocybe Fanaticus" PF Tek method, that revolutionized the cultivation of mushrooms indoors. Vermiculite's addition to an underlying basis for a grain substrate (rather than just using grains alone) was the key innovation of McPherson that gave the mycelium more space to grow and mimicking the natural environment. While his method is more labor intensive than other approaches and yields less however, it's a great choice for beginners due to its ease of use as well as its low cost and reliability. Additionally, it utilizes materials and products which are readily available, and many of them are already in your home.

SYRINGES SPORE

A nice spore syringe could be one thing you might find difficult to locate. It can hold your magical mushroom spores until they "sow" them in the soil. Incorrect strains, contamination, as well as syringes with just water have been reported by some growers. There shouldn't be any issues when you conduct your research and find a trustworthy supplier. After you've harvested the first lot (or flush) of mushrooms, you'll be able to begin filling your own Syringes.

What you'll need

In order to begin you'll require some things, but don't be concerned it only needs to be purchased once and it will cost you less over the long term compared to purchasing a grow kit or purchasing by the grams.

INGREDIENTS

* 10-12 cc sporesyringe

* Rice flour from brown (organic)

* Medium/fine vermiculite

* Drinking water

Equipment

12-half-pint shoulderless shoulderless jars without lids (e.g. ball or Kerr jelly or canning containers)

* A small nail, and Hammer

* Cup to measure

* Bowl to mix

* Strainer

* Tin foil (heavy-duty)

* To steam it is necessary to use a large cookware with a secure lid is needed.

* Small towel (or approximately. 10-paper towels)

* Tape that has micropores

The clear storage bin

You can use a drill with a diameter of 14 inches for drill.

* Perlite

* Spray bottle to mist

SUPPLIES FOR HYGIENE

* Rubs alcohol onto

* Torch lighter (butane/propane)

* Disinfectant that can be used for surfaces.

* Sanitizer to clean the air

The gloves are sterilized (optional)

* Mask for Surgical Surgery (optional)

* A quiet room or a glove box (optional)

Chapter 6: Health Mushroom Benefits

THERE ARE SEVERAL POTENTIAL BENEFITS THAT CAN DERIVED FROM THE CONSUMPTION OF MAGIC MUSHROOM, RANGING FROM THE TREATMENT OF DEPRESSION TO HELPING MANAGE ALCOHOL ADDICTION BUT NONE HAVE YET TO BE APPROVED BY THE FDA. In addition to STEREOTYPES and testing various PSYCHEDELIC MUSHROOMS SCIENTIFIC researchers are on the increase to determine if there any effect on the treatment of MYRIAD-related psychiatric disorders that include depression as well as anxiety. They have been promising results over the past decade.

MAGIC Mushrooms can be consumed either in their raw form or with beverages, OR INTRAVENOUS Injures. After her oral intake, PSILOCYBIN RAPIDLY METABOLIZES IN the liver, and then transforms into the active form PSILOCIN and is then absorbed by the blood stream and circulates down until it reaches the BRAIN. When it reaches the BRAIN, it is bound to neurochemical RECEPTORS known as SEROTONIN RECEPTORS. These receptors are located in the

BRAIN and are housed BY NEURONS , which, upon activation, trigger an increase in the activity of the BRAIN which can be reflected in memory and MOOD BEHAVIOUR and emotions.

At the beginning, Psilocybin containing mushrooms were intended to be used to treat psychotherapeutic issues. However, due to the growing popularity of recreational use in the general population the use of her medicinal properties was banned in the year 1970. In the 30th year of suspension however, the use of Psilocybin was once again permitted to be used for research. At present, there is some doubts regarding the legality of Psilocybin. For certain countries, such as UK and USA There is a certain amount of ban on using Psilocybin and in other nations, such as the majority of Europe and Australia It is completely illegal. Therefore, it is crucial to verify the legality of the magic mushroom within the country you live in.

Lowers Depression

After a couple of administrations Psilocybin has been proven to be effective in treating depression in those suffering from cancer and with treatment-resistant depression. The researchers of the Center for Psychedelic and Consciousness Research at Johns Hopkins Bay view Medical Center located in Baltimore, Maryland, evaluated the effects of psilocybin for people aged between 21 and 75 years who suffer from major depressive disorder in a controlled clinical trial that was published within JAMA (MDD). These patients were not taking antidepressants, and were not suffering from a depression, major suicide attempts or hospitalization. 24 patients received two treatments with psilocybin (session 1 20 mg/70 kg and sessions 2 and 3:30 mg/70kg) in addition to about 11 hours of support psychotherapy in the study.

The authors said, "The results of this randomized clinical study demonstrated the effectiveness of psilocybin-assisted treatment in delivering large, rapid and lasting antidepressant benefits for patients suffering from MDD." "These results are in line with the results of previous trials that included patients with depression and cancer and also those with treatment-resistant depression. This suggests that psilocybin might be effective in a much larger group that includes MDD people." Further research doing active treatment or placebo-controlled treatments and with larger and more diverse populations is required."

Helps to Form New brain cells.

As per research psilocybin in mushrooms helps in the creation of brain cells that are new. It assists in the brain's ability to conquer anxiety and boosts the growth of neurons which results in the regenerative neurons in our brains. The brain gets more active because of the increase in brain cells. It also develops the capacity to remember learn, recall, and remember specific actions. This reduces the chance of harmful stimuli damaging brain cells.

Mysterious Mushrooms and Pain

There is an increasing research base about magical mushrooms, specifically for mental health issues. The FDA declared psilocybin one of the most effective therapies in the year 2018. Then there was the Psychedelics and Health Research Initiative (PHRI) located at UC San Diego was established with the intention of studying the effects of psilocybin along with similar substances to help in reducing pain and speed up healing.

In an upcoming BMJ study, PHRI researchers focused on the potential benefits of psilocybin as well as other psychedelics to help in the treatment of pain.

"Psychedelics can alter your mind's perception. This has been proven to reset functional connectivity (FC) within the brain. These regions are key to many neuropathic conditions in the central nervous system as per serotonin 2A (5-HT2A) receptor agonism." In comparison to opioid analgesics, psychedelics generally have a positive safety assessment. "Although there is a lack of evidence from clinical studies for their usage for chronic pain, numerous studies and reports released over the past 50 years have shown the potential for analgesic effects in cancer pain as well as phantom limb pain and cluster headaches," they said.

"Abnormalities in FC caused by psychedelics suggest that these medications could be able to reverse the neural connections observed in chronic pain." They said that in light of the current epidemic of opioids and the limited effectiveness of non-opioid analgesics investigation into psychedelics' analgesics is required to improve the lives of those suffering from chronic pain.

Quitting smoking and overcoming other addictions

Certain people lead unhealthy lives and have a hard time maintaining their effectiveness through following the right way. The prevalence of addiction is all around us and it is difficult to get rid of. Mushrooms on the other side, are helpful in treating addiction. They are used for treating chemical addictions like cocaine and nicotine. Researchers investigated the use of the psychotherapy of psilocybin in helping addicts overcome their dependence on harmful substances in a research.

Addiction can lead to an euphoria state where we are unable to think, ask questions and develop healthily. It weakens and dulls your ability to live a healthy life. The mushroom has proven that they are extremely helpful for mankind, since they have the ability to be used to treat certain of the most serious diseases, like addiction.'

More "Openness" along with other positive Personality Changes

We are born in freedom without ties, and full with compassion. These qualities allow us to grow, learn and be connected as sentient beings. Researchers have discovered that mushrooms assist us in being more open to others, develop and develop in accordance with a study. Significant increases in openness after high-dose psilocybin sessions according to researchers. It is a trait that shows a person's attitude towards new experiences. It may also help in developing their imagination, creativity and appreciation for creativity. The effects of the mushrooms on human nature openness can last over an entire year. In the end, mushrooms are able to help improve the harmony between human natural environment and the surrounding.

Helps you to break free of the Ego and boost your creativity.

As we've mentioned the mushrooms provide a myriad of benefits for health. They aid us in growing in our health, living a balanced lifestyle and fighting depression. The mushrooms, on their own, help us deal with our self-image. One of the main causes of inflexibility and temperament issues is the human self-image. It is nothing but the assertion of your superiority over other people. The mushrooms, in contrast aid us in dealing with our egos, and also give us the capacity to be more imaginative. The development of new ideas is the result of creativity which helps you succeed. It's not recommended to have an attitude of ego toward anyone, particularly when working in any industry. When we've overcome our self-esteem then we'll be able open a new chapter in our lives and feel more alive.

Chapter 7: Effects Of Magic Mushrooms

"The most frequent consequence of using psilocybin is a feeling of anxiety. It can vary from a "bad trip or a debilitating hallucination that can last for several weeks "American Addiction Centers chief medical officer Dr. Lawrence Weinstein, told Insight.

The mind-altering effects of psilocybin-containing mushrooms normally last six to eight hours under normal conditions, depending on dosage, preparation method, and personal metabolism. The most intense phase of this period typically occurs in the first three or four hours. Due to the fact that psilocybin can alter perception of time, the effects may appear to last longer for the user, as per the Dr. Weinstein.

Your experience experiencing the magic mushrooms is affected by a myriad of elements, including the dose of the environment, the people you're in with, and also your mood or state of mind before you consume the mushrooms. Feeling anxious or depressed prior to the consumption of psilocybin may intensify any negative feelings you experience, leading to an unpleasant experience.

People suffering with mental illness or mood issues should consider taking in mushrooms that are magical. Consuming mushrooms can have negative consequences for those who's mental health is affected by the way psilocybin works on the brain. "Psilocin's relationship with serotonin receptors within the prefrontal cortex may alter the brain's chemical composition, making disorders such as bipolar disorder, panic disorder disorders, and anxiety more severe," Dr. Weinstein explained. Even people who do not have a family history of mental illness could experience an increase in anxiety attacks after the use of magical mushrooms.

Doctor. Cali Estes, Ph.D. Addiction specialist and the founder of The Addictions Academy, told INSIDER, "When the mushrooms affect your system, they expose you to the risk of panic or extreme anxiety events, such as dizziness and lightheadedness."

There is evidence that taking magical mushrooms under the guidance by a doctor may help with anxiety, although more studies are needed.

Since magic mushrooms are considered illegal in a majority of countries and not restricted like other substances It's difficult to determine the exact results you'll get if you purchase a bag. "Some magical mushrooms are actually the same mushrooms that are sold in stores, but with a different hallucinogen such as PCP or LSD or a completely new drug," the doctor. Weinstein cautioned.

The purchase of magic mushrooms could put you in risk of consuming a range of other substances that could result in a fatal overdose or adverse reaction. You should avoid taking a psilocybin supplement when you're not sure about its authenticity.

One of the most dangerous scenarios with regard to magical mushrooms is consuming poisonous mushrooms instead of one with the psilocybin. People who attempt to gather their own mushrooms outdoors, as per the Dr. Weinstein, are more susceptible to poisoning by harmful

169

species because it's easy to mistake the fungus that is dangerous with the hallucinogenic mushrooms. Insomnia, weakness in the muscle stomach problems as well as delirium, are signs of poisoning from mushrooms and should be treated by a doctor immediately when you suspect you've eaten a dangerous mushroom.

It's a popular myth that there's no risk of taking too much magical mushrooms. It's not true however. "It is possible to overdose on mushrooms, but it's not common. Paranoia, panic attacks, anxiety, psychosis, vomiting and seizures are just a few signs of an overdose on mushrooms "Dr. Weinstein stated.

"The consequences of eating 'too many mushrooms' last between 6-8 hour," Dr. Weinstein added, "although some of the symptoms can take several days to disappear." If you accidentally consume more psilocybin than anticipated and you experience adverse reactions, seeking medical attention is the best choice.

It is possible that psychedelic substances such as magic mushrooms could trigger psychosis.

However, recent research in controlled environments have revealed no connection between the substances and the growth of psychosis. "Psychosis that is caused by psilocybin which is remarkably like schizophrenia, could be caused through the use of psychedelic substances. Psychotic episodes are more likely in those who have a history of family members of schizophrenia or any other psychotic disorder "Dr. Weinstein stated.

If someone has had a large amount of psilocybin, or other mushrooms is more likely to suffer this serious negative result. "Depending on the quantity and frequency of consumption and frequency, magic mushrooms can cause lasting neurological damage" Dr. Estes stated. The consumption of magic mushrooms has been shown to affect permanently the brain, but it isn't always believed to be a problem.

A different, but potentially dangerous adverse effect that can be a result associated with psychedelic fungi is the creation of HPPD which is a hallucinogen-induced chronic perception disorder. "Even even if one does not take the substance, HPPD can cause a person to experience flashbacks of their experiences being under the effects of hallucinogens weeks, days, or even years following their last use. The disease may cause someone to experience frightening hallucinations and great stress "Dr. Weinstein forewarned.

Being afflicted by other mental health issues or using hallucinogens regularly for a long duration are potential risk factors for developing this illness. The condition, however, has no official treatment.

The hallucinations, and the sense of altered real-world reality magic mushrooms give are typically embraced by users. This altered view of the world however is able to motivate people to take risky risks or to put themselves in danger without realizing it.

The consumption of mushrooms can make you more vulnerable to harm by affecting your judgement and causing sleepiness, confusion and loss of motor coordination. But, there are no studies that have been conducted to establish the connection between the use of recreational mushrooms and risky behavior.

There's nothing in magical mushrooms that could cause chemical addictionlike it is with heroin or nicotine. However, mushrooms do can create problems in your life , if they cause you to lose focus or avoid other pursuits or obligations. "Someone who spends more time contemplating them, not doing work in order to gain a high and/or consuming excessively or intoxicated mushrooms regularly are all signs of addiction" stated the Dr. Estes. Dr. Weinstein, on the contrary, emphasized that there isn't any evidence that proves the fact that mushrooms and other psychedelic substances are addictive physically or mentally.

It is possible that you will become less susceptible to other mind-altering substances if you use the magic mushrooms regularly on a daily routine. "Continual use of these mushrooms can cause people to develop the condition of a cross-tolerance. That is, they'll develop a strong tolerance to similar substances like LSD or marijuana" the doctor. Weinstein stated. Since it is impossible to determine the degree of strength that uncontrolled substances such as marijuana and LSD are, establishing the cross-tolerance could put you at the risk to take too high other psychoactive drugs to experience the full effects.

MOSHROOM POISONING

The poisoning of mushrooms, also known as toadstool poisoning is a deadly, and sometimes fatal, result from eating toxic mushrooms (toadstools). There are between 70 and 80 kinds of mushrooms that can be poisonous to humans. Many contain harmful alkaloids (muscarine and agaricine as well as and phalline).

The most frequently cause poisoning is Amanita Muscaria Amanita phalloides, as well as those four white Amanita species known as the destroying angels. Ingestion of Amanita Muscaria (fly agaric) is a muscarine-rich mushroom. as well as other alkaloids that can cause poisoning, is followed by vomiting, nausea, diarrhea and excessive sweating as well as eye watering slow and difficult breathing, pupils that are dilated and confusion. It can also cause excitation and confusion. The symptoms usually begin in the first few hours following eating the mushrooms. Recovery generally happens within 12 hours.

Amanita phalloides, also known as the death cap, also known as the death cup, is much more deadly than the muscarine variety It contains heat-stable peptide poisons, phalloidin, as well as two amanitins that harm cell membranes throughout our body. In the 6-12 hours of eating the mushrooms intense abdominal pain nausea, vomiting, as well as bloody diarrhea are common, leading to rapid loss of fluids from the tissues as well as extreme thirst. The signs of a severe involvement of the kidneys, the liver along with the central nervous system show up, including decreased urinary output and a decrease in blood sugar. The condition can lead to the condition of coma that, in more than 50 % instances, ends in the death.

This variety Gyromitra (Helvella) has an endocrine that is normally eliminated during cooking, however certain people are vulnerable to it. The chemical composition of the toxin is not been identified, however, it's a source for monomethylhydrazine. It is a neurotoxic agent that affects the nervous system of central nerves, and can cause hemolytic jaundice.

Some patients suffering from severe Amanita poisoning are successfully treated with the combination of thioctic acids as well as glucose and penicillin, or by passing blood through an charcoal filter. The best way to prevent it is to steer clear of consuming any wild mushrooms that have not been identified in a qualified authority.

HOW to store and harvest mushrooms

IN MOST CASES IT IS VERY DIFFICULT TO KNOW WHEN YOU CAN HARVEST YOUR MUSHROOMS IN YOUR GROW KIT. Sometimes, it's easier if all the mushrooms were the same size and could be harvested at once, but This isn't the scenario. When your MUSHROOMS have grown large ENOUGH to warrant a harvest, there is usually a large number of smaller and medium-sized MUSHROOMS which may still be able to grow a bit more among them. A common MISTAKE the majority of PEOPLE make is to remove the larger

MUSHROOMS first so that the smaller and medium-sized mushrooms can continue to grow. This MISTAKE UNKNOWN to many people who grow mushrooms will not raise the yield, but, more importantly it could result in contamination of your grow kit.

Watch for FRUITS: After 5 to 12 days, your mushrooms are ready to harvest. First, your MUSHROOM or FRUITS, will appear as tiny white bumps before being pushed into "PINS."

Pick your favorite fruits: Cut your mushrooms close to the CAKE and then remove them once they are ready for harvest. Do not allow them to get to the point of no return in their Growth, mainly because when they mature, they will begin to lose their potenency.

Note: The ideal moment to collect your mushrooms is before the veil begins to break. If it is at this point, your fungus will be conical in shape with light caps, as well as gills covered with a tarp.

STORING Mushrooms

In the refrigerator the psilocybin mushroom will usually become stale after a couple of weeks. If you're planning to utilize them for microdosing or just keep them in the future you'll have to think about storage. Drying is the most efficient method to store them for the long term. So long as they're kept in a dark, cold and dry place They should last for between two and three years. They'll last almost forever as long as they're kept stored in the freezer.

The idea of letting your mushrooms dry on a paper sheet for a few days perhaps even in the shade of a fan is a simple method to dry the mushrooms. The problem with this method is that they'll always ever "cracker dry." This means that they won't snap when you attempt at bending them. which allows them to keep water. Based on the length of time you let them sit you can decrease in energy. The most effective method is to make use of the dehydrator, but these aren't cheap. Utilizing a desiccant such as the following is a good alternative

Dry your mushrooms for up to 48 to 72 hours outdoors, best using a blower.

* Fill the bottom of the container using desiccant. Desiccants accessible include silica gel kitty litter as well as anhydrous calcium chloride both are available at hardware shops.

Cover the desiccant using wire racks or similar to prevent the mushrooms from getting close to it.

Then, arrange your mushrooms in the rack. Then close the container to ensure the mushrooms aren't too close.

* After a couple of days, make sure to check the dryness of your clothes.

* Transfer to freezer-safe storage containers (e.g. Ziploc, vacuum-sealed).

MICRODOSING

It is crucial to follow the right dosage for any medication. A doctor might prescribe 1000mg of antibiotics every day for two days to combat an infection caused by bacteria. This is exactly the dosage the patient needs to consume. It is essential to do the same procedure when taking supplements enhancements like psilocybin mushrooms.

Many people take drugs, like the psilocybin fungus, recreationally frequently. It causes them to drink excessive quantities, which causes toxic effects in the brain as well as the body. It also increases the firing of neuronal cells in the central nervous system. The risk of overdose is low, but the psilocybin mushroom can be fatal. A study of more than 12,000 users of the psilocybin fungus discovered that just 0.2 percent needed medical attention.

Microdosing is the most effective way to take advantage of the benefits of these mushrooms. It has many advantages and lower the risk of suffering adverse side effects.

What is the benefit of microdosing instead of taking the full dose?

Microdosing refers to the deliberate use tiny amounts of psychedelic compounds that are not enough to experience hallucinogenic results. While this practice is expanding in popularity, it's still under-studied. Although the microdosing of hallucinogenic chemicals has seen a rise in popularity over the past 10 years The most important question is whether or not it will produce positive effects on the mind.

If microdosing, or taking the full dosage of a medication is the most effective option is still a debate. Psychonauts might think that treatment using full doses of psilocybin is the most effective method to treat mental disorders such as clinical depression and PTSD.

Microdosing is the most effective method to get psilocybin mushrooms. Microdosing is a smaller amount than is required for a high. Microdosing does not have a predetermined quantity. Every person is unique and therefore there could be different doses. Many people believe that microdosing should be less than a tenth of typical dose (approximately 0.01 to 0.3 grams of the psilocybin mushrooms). This is the primary controversy surrounding microdosing. People who oppose it believe that microdosing ultimately leads to tolerance which could require greater doses over time.

Although there is a possibility of tolerance in the case of regular use of psilocybin Studies have demonstrated that microdosing the psilocybin mushroom for long periods of time can lower depression and anxiety. There have been some instances of people being emotionally overwhelmed from prolonged usage, the majority of cases were positive.

Microdosing The Benefits and Challenges of Microdosing

Although research on microdosing have been very limited There are numerous personal accounts of individuals who have utilized online forums to share their experiences this method. Microdosing can dramatically improve mood. People who use microdoses report feeling less anxious as well as more optimistic and depressed. More than 80% respondents report feeling happier. People with a positive outlook on life could manage more serious mental illnesses like PTSD or clinical depression for shorter durations.

A lot of people have reported a similar benefit: they were more focused in their work and were more successful at their work. Many reported an improvement in efficiency and creativity, as well as empathy and teamwork. While there are some risks with psilocybin however, those who take it prudently can reap the long-term advantages.

Microdosing may have numerous benefits However, it also comes with its drawbacks. It is recommended to buy these items legally. Psilocybin mushrooms are banned in numerous countries. It may be challenging to obtain them without violating any laws.

How do you prepare and take your microdosing

To alter your microdosing regimen it is essential to pay attention at your body. You must be attentive and cautious for you to enjoy the benefits of microdosing psilocybin mushroom. Before you are able to consume the mushrooms, it is crucial to be aware of the amount.

It is necessary to limit the amount of mushrooms that you consume fresh. This is due to the fact that they decrease in their power. Because they are easy to store, the majority times dried mushrooms are the best choice. It is possible to adjust the dosage in accordance with your personal preferences.

* Do not consume less than 0.1 grams of mushrooms for each person when you weigh below 130 lbs.

* You can increase the serving size of 0.2 grams for each serving when you weigh between 130 and 180 pounds.

The amount can be increased to 0.3 grams for each serving when you weigh more than 180 pounds.

Microdosing could be beneficial for creative people and is a great option for graphic designers.

There are a variety of ways to consume mushrooms. Some are more exotic than others, while others are fairly easy. This article outlines the five top techniques. Pick the method that is most appealing and relevant to you.